STUTTERING and what you can do about it

by WENDELL JOHNSON

UNIVERSITY OF MINNESOTA PRESS

MINNEAPOLIS

TO ALL THE OLDSTERS AND YOUNGSTERS
AND THEIR PARENTS
WITH, ABOUT, AND FOR WHOM THIS BOOK
HAS BEEN WRITTEN

With Appreciation and Best Wishes

THIS book is for parents who are afraid their children are going to grow up to be stutterers, for speakers who have grown up to be stutterers, and for all who see in stuttering one of the most interesting and distinctively human of the quandaries of man.

It is a hopeful book. It is based on scientific research findings. It is designed to be helpful.

Much of this book deals with the relation of parents to the problem of stuttering. In introducing the pages that lie ahead, I want to say a few friendly words of reassurance to you who are parents. We are often told that the trouble with children is parents. I, for one, think this view is neither fair nor scientifically sound. There are many factors besides parents that affect the lives of the young in our society. There are doctors, teachers, preachers, and publishers; television, radio, and neighborhood gossip; the corner drugstore, the skating rink, the recreation center, and the city playground; to say nothing of climate, cold germs, cost of living, food fads, and books on child psychology — and speech pathology.

When all has been said and pondered, it is only fair to consider that parents have had parents too. And their parents had parents. The particular generation of mothers and fathers who are now striving to cope with the hazards and the distracting joys of bringing up their own children are not to be blamed for all the folly that has come down through the ages, any more than they are to be credited with all the wisdom abroad in the world today.

When parents are made to feel guilty and uneasy by being blamed for the mistakes and miseries of their children, matters tend to be made worse instead of better. The distress which they and their children share is complicated and deepened. The plain truth is that very often it is the blaming itself that is to blame when things go wrong or worsen.

It is something else again to face up to facts. This has nothing to do with blaming anybody. It is helpful, of course, to parents as well as to their youngsters, and to those who serve their special needs, to have clear descriptions of the difficulties children and parents do have with each other. It is worthwhile, therefore, to observe with care and report in detail the problems that arise in the interactions between parents and children, and to explain them in ways that suggest practical solutions.

It is in such a spirit that this book has been written for you who are parents and for its other readers as well.

You have every right to be hopeful if stuttering is your problem — or your child's problem. Methods of dealing with stuttering, and of preventing it, have been greatly improved in recent years. With continuing research, and proper education of young parents and of the general public, we may all but eliminate the problem in the years ahead.

In the meantime, there is much information that can be helpful to you. You stand to gain particularly from knowing about the way the problem arises in specific cases — in cases more or less like your own. The better you understand the way the problem begins — its causes, that is — the more you can do to prevent it in the first place, or to keep it from developing further once it has arisen, or to deal with it effectively if it is already well developed.

What is known about the problem called stuttering can be put in few words or many, and both the many and the few — detailed accounts and brief summaries — are to be found in this book. In general, the book is made up of statements of information, of explanation, and of practical application. Since it has been written especially for the parents and the youthful and adult stutterers who have practical reasons for reading it, it is designed to contain enough factual information to make the explanations and recommendations — and summaries — meaningful and useful.

Readers who desire additional information are referred to the following books, upon which this one is largely based: *Stuttering in Children and Adults: Thirty Years of Research at the University of Iowa*, edited by Wendell Johnson with the assistance of Ralph Leutenegger (Minneapolis: University of Minnesota Press, 1955; 472 pp.); *The Onset of Stuttering: Research Findings and Implications*, by Wendell Johnson and Associates (Minneapolis: University of Minnesota Press, 1959; 519 pp.). "Toward Understanding Stuttering," which I prepared in 1959 for the National Society for Crippled Children and Adults, 2023 West Ogden Avenue, Chicago 10, Illinois, is a companion pamphlet, for parents, based on *The Onset of Stuttering*. "An Open Letter to the Mother of a Stuttering Child," a small pamphlet also based on the Iowa stuttering research findings, is published by the Interstate Printers and Publishers, Danville, Illinois.

Parts of this book are based on other technical publications, most important of which are relevant research and clinical reports in the *Journal of Speech and Hearing Disorders* and the *Journal of Speech and Hearing Research*, published quarterly by the American Speech and Hearing Association, 1001 Connecticut Avenue N.W., Washington 6, D.C. Of particular interest in relation to certain passages in Chapter 10 is *The Problem of Stuttering in Certain North American Indian Societies*, by Joseph Stewart, Monograph Supplement 6, *Journal of Speech and Hearing Disorders*, 1960. A considerable body of pertinent research data is to be found in *Studies of Speech Fluency and Disfluency in Stutterers and Nonstutterers*, by Wendell Johnson and Associates, Monograph Supplement 7, *Journal of Speech and Hearing Disorders*, 1961.

I should like to explain that the lovable and noble physician who played the role of Dr. Gregory in "Toward Understanding Stuttering" returns in Chapter 1 of this book bearing his real name, Dr. Hedinger. Dr. Hedinger's town in Kansas, which was named Crayton in the earlier publication, is here referred to by its official name of Canton. The town of Roxbury is identified by its real name in both accounts.

The parents who participated in the clinical studies underlying this book are deserving of the thanks of all those who may find value in its pages. The stutterers who have helped in the laboratory and clinic to deepen our understanding of the problem they share have also earned our gratitude. I am personally mindful of the assistance and companionship in my own research and clinical activities of a large company of friends and associates, many of whom I have mentioned in introductions to previously published books and research reports. Individual acknowledgments here beyond the few which follow are hardly feasible, but to all who know that I mean them, my warmest thanks.

I was persuaded to undertake this book by Mr. A. A. Heckman, executive director of the Louis W. and Maud Hill Family Foundation, and I was generously encouraged and ably counseled in the planning of it by Mr. John Ervin, Jr., director, and Miss Jeanne Sinnen, senior editor, of the University of Minnesota Press. The technical counsel of Miss Janet Salisbury of the publishing staff was also of great value. The services of Mr. Charles Burns, literary and publishing consultant, have been extremely helpful and I am very grateful for them. I should like to record, too, that Chapters 10 and 11 reflect the evaluative readings made of them in manuscript form by Professor Dean Williams and W. Hugh Missildine, M.D. My warm thanks reflect my conviction that this book is much the better for the influence of these friends and counselors, but my thanks by no means imply that they are to be held accountable for any of the book's shortcomings, for which I am alone responsible.

A major proportion of the research that has made the book possible was completed under a series of grants from the Louis W. and Maud Hill Family Foundation. The research program is being carried forward under additional grants from the Foundation and also from the Federal Office of Vocational Rehabilitation. Supplementary funds have been granted by the Easter Seal Foundation of the National Society for Crippled Children and Adults. Basic institutional support for the total laboratory and clinical program has long been provided by the University of Iowa. It is scarcely possible to express adequately the deep sense of appreciation with which I acknowledge the support that my associates and I have been given in carrying on our studies of stuttering.

WITH APPRECIATION AND BEST WISHES

Mrs. Shirley Dunn and Miss Margaret Seemuth typed the several drafts of the manuscript, and Miss Ruth Farstrup assisted in reading proof and making the index. I am appreciative of their patience and competence.

My most perceptive and resilient literary critic is my wife, whose readings and re-readings of the book in manuscript form resulted, fortunately for its readers, in many of the major and the finely detailed revisions involved in its several redraftings.

For more than half a century the presidents and other administrative officers of the University of Iowa, representing the citizens of the state, have encouraged scientific and humanitarian work in the interests of children and adults with problems of speech and hearing. On behalf of all who share my sense of gratitude for this benevolent tradition and for the continuing enlightened interest and support of President Virgil M. Hancher and his administrative associates, I am deeply pleased to express warm appreciation.

WENDELL JOHNSON

Iowa City, Iowa
March 8, 1960

Table of Contents

STUTTERING

and what you can do about it

CHAPTER 1

In Search of Beginnings and Endings

My REASONS for wanting to understand the problem called stuttering were, and are, reasons like yours, if stuttering is your own or your child's problem. It was not that I intended, when I started, to go deeply into the subject. On the contrary, I only wanted to "have my stuttering cured."

It all started when I was quite small, but even so I didn't always have the problem. I remember going when I was five with my sister to her school in Roxbury two miles from our farm in Kansas. It was a large frame building painted white and to me the door was enormous. I walked through it and seemed immediately to be standing beside the teacher's desk and I had almost to reach up a little to place my hand on top of it. The teacher seemed large to me and her face was round, and I liked looking at it. I started to speak a piece while I was still looking at the teacher with my back to the children. I heard them laughing, and the teacher told me to turn around and speak my piece to them. They seemed to fill the room as I looked at them and said:

> I asked my mother for fifty cents
> To see the elephant jump the fence.
> He jumped so high he hit the sky
> And didn't come down till the Fourth of July.

They all sat still and listened, and though I can't remember what they did after that, my memory of the day is pleasant. My family, I've been told, and maybe others too, thought I spoke well, and so I was taken to school to speak a piece — and apparently acquitted myself satisfactorily.

The next thing I remember about speaking was when I was six,

3

and I had started going to school. I went to school in the same big white building where I had spoken my piece about the elephant the year before, and to the same nice teacher who had said I should look at the children while I spoke. After I had been going to school for a month or two she came to our home one evening, or maybe it was a Sunday afternoon, and talked to my mother and father.

She told them she had thought some of moving me ahead to the second grade soon after I started school but, she said, I was beginning to stutter, and so she had decided to keep me in the first grade. I don't know whether she said they should do something about my speech or not. Although they had never thought there was any-thing the matter with my speech until the teacher talked to them about it, they must have taken her word for it that something was the matter, and I have no evidence they ever asked her what she meant by "stuttering." I don't suppose she ever wondered much herself about what she meant.

I remember vividly the astonishment with which I suddenly realized, one day about twenty-five years ago, that apparently for a month or so the teacher had been the only person who had thought I was stuttering. I had been talking during that month, and before of course, to my parents and my brothers and sisters, and the other children at school, and the man at the general store, and lots of other people — and none of them had said, or thought, as far as I have been able to find out, that I was stuttering. Whatever the teacher was talking about, none of them had noticed it, or if they had they hadn't thought of it as stuttering.

Having taken the teacher's word for it that I was beginning to stutter, my parents did what many other parents would have done under the circumstances. They took me — not at once but after some time had passed — to the doctor. In our case "the doctor" was not just another physician, not to us at any rate. He was a very special sort of person, and I would understand after many years that he had been in his own way the Albert Schweitzer of our little valley. I remember, as though from a world that no longer exists, that day, nearly a half-century ago, when I sat beside my father on the tufted black leather buggy seat, weaving wisps of childish wonder to the cadence of the horses' hooves along the gently rolling ten miles to old Doctor Hedinger's office in Canton.

The French people were still talking of the possible return from exile, once again, of the Emperor Napoleon Bonaparte when Doctor Hedinger was born. He had been a contemporary of Lincoln and Lee, and he had outlived most of his contemporaries when Alexander Graham Bell invented the telephone in 1876. Doctor Hedinger's era had passed into history long before he died one day from eating too much boiled cabbage, it was said, at the age of 97. He is etched in my memory as though he were a cameo, leaning toward me slightly with his full-length black coat draped like a toga from his thin shoulders. From his narrow bronzed face his white beard extended to his waistband and he seemed to hover over me like Father Time himself as he asked me with a twinkle in his eyes to say "Philadelphia."

I cannot be certain whether I passed this first of many, many speech tests the years were to hold for me, but I was never to be tested by a wiser examiner. Doctor Hedinger was so very wise that he knew the depths of his own ignorance. I know now that no one knew very much about the problem called stuttering in those days, and that old Doctor Hedinger was probably as well — or meagerly — informed about it as anyone else within a thousand, or even ten thousand, miles of Canton. But what he lacked in scientific knowledge he made up in sensitivity. He understood, Doctor Hedinger did, that it is precisely at those times when nothing can be done that it is most essential that one do something, and something as nice as possible. And so he gave me a pretty little bottle of sugar pills. But, being kind as well as wise, he flavored the pills with peppermint.

One of the pictures of my mother that is clear in my memory is of her standing that evening after supper by the cupboard, holding my little bottle of peppermint pills to her nose, her brown eyes narrowed in thoughtful disbelief.

Those peppermint pills were to become for me in later years a very powerful symbol — of love without understanding. If, in 1912, Congress had appropriated a million dollars for the stutterers, young and old, of this country, the money would have been spent, of neces-

5

sity, for sugar pills, or their equivalent — with or without pepper-mint depending upon the public demands for economy. That something more effective can be done today is to be explained by the fact that in the meantime the problem of stuttering has been taken into the laboratory and subjected to scientific study.

◀ ◀ ◀

All through my school years my father persisted in trying to find someone who could "do something about my stuttering," or some method by which he could help me or I could help myself. He read one day in the paper that stutterers could talk by holding their teeth together, and so this I tried, but my father was a man of sound practical judgment and I did not talk in this strange fashion for long. By the time I had emerged from the tenderest years of childhood our family had acquired an automobile, and I remember a day when I was ten or twelve being driven with my father to Wichita, sixty miles away, to see a college professor there "who used to stutter." In slow and measured tones, he advised me to breathe in "with the diaphragm" before speaking and to exhale slowly while I spoke. This seemed pretty much like being advised to walk across the street by putting one foot ahead of the other — and it must not have made much difference in the way I talked, because soon after that my father took me to another man, an itinerant preacher of considerable reputation in those parts, who admonished me to have faith and to use great determination. He assured me I could do anything I thought I could.

Whether he was mistaken or I was lacking in determination I can't be sure, I suppose, but at any rate the next stop on my tour of hope and desperation was a little town in the Missouri Ozarks, to which my father was attracted while on a business trip by word that there was a healer of sorts who held forth there. The ride through the flint hills of southeastern Kansas and into the beautiful Ozarks was pleasant enough, but my memory of the alleged healer is extremely obscure. I recall dimly that he talked to us about his "electrical machines," and I suspect my father's patience gave out rather quickly. I shall never forget, though, how astonished I was a few hours later at dusk in Springfield by the bareheaded and barefooted, white-robed and white-bearded old man of the mountain who carried a long staff and prophesied in a high tremulous voice to all who cared to pause and heed that the end of the world was near, at least in Springfield, Missouri. But the end of neither the world nor my stuttering came to pass.

When my father read the story of Demosthenes, who, as a rather erroneous but inspiring legend has it, overcame a speech impediment by standing on the seashore with pebbles under his tongue and shouting above the roar of the waves, to become the greatest orator of ancient Greece, I talked for several days with pebbles, as well as BB shot and other things, under my tongue. No results were apparent, however, at least up to the time my father's will to experiment was overcome by my mother's fear that I would swallow something that would have to be removed by surgery.

A summer of adjustments by a chiropractor having failed to loosen my tongue, my father was next persuaded, against his better judgment, by my innocent faith in a newspaper advertisement which guaranteed to cure my stuttering, "or your money back," to allow me to go away to a "stuttering school." I was sixteen. It was my first train ride, my first venture east of the Mississippi, my first visit alone to a big city — and my first profoundly unnerving disappointment. It was also perhaps my first major lesson in semantics, from which I learned far more than I could possibly comprehend at the time about the meanings of words such as "guarantee" and "cure" and "money back." After three months of speaking with a very extreme drawl, reading aloud in dirge time, and swinging dumbbells while chanting, one word to a swing, "Have more backbone and less wishbone" and "Little drops of water will wear away a rock," I returned home more hesitant and tense in speech than ever, and so thoroughly demoralized it didn't even occur to me to try to get my money back.

Some three years later when I was a sophomore in McPherson College in Kansas, I learned that a program of research on stuttering was being started at the University of Iowa in Iowa City. After an exchange of letters with Lee Edward Travis, a professor in the departments of psychology, speech, and psychiatry at the university

7

who was in charge of the program, I made my way in the fall of 1926 to Iowa City.

A few days after I arrived Dr. Travis asked me to come with him to one of his classes. He explained that he wanted the students to observe my speech. I sat in a chair beside his desk at the front of the room. There were thirty or forty students looking at me. Dr. Travis told them who I was and that I was from a small town in Kansas, and then he handed me a book and asked me to read aloud to the students. I read for five minutes — and got out four words.

After class I went with him to his car and we got in and started for the other end of the campus. When we had gone about a block he stopped to give one of the staff members a ride, and as she got in the car he introduced us. Then he started the car again and we drove down a long curving hill and crossed a river. A couple hundred yards beyond the river we turned a corner, went a block, turned another corner and went up another hill. Altogether we had gone about a mile when all of a sudden I finally managed to blurt out, "Puhleased to meet you!" They were startled, and so was I, and I wished I hadn't said it, only I would have been even more embarrassed if I hadn't said anything at all.

That year I stretched my six feet two inches the full length of a couch in Dr. Travis' office nearly every day for an hour, talking as fast and as freely as I could about anything and everything that oozed and bubbled up out of the lower caverns of my consciousness or "my unconscious" or early childhood, or wherever it came from, while Dr. Travis sat behind a screen a few feet beyond the back of my head and made notes. I stuttered a lot. I mean I tightened up the muscles I used in talking and held my breath now and then for a long time, while trying hard to speak in spite of the things I was doing which, as I realize now, made speaking impossible or nearly so. What I remember most clearly about how I felt is that I didn't like the way I felt, and my tensions and strain in talking were almost completely mysterious to me. I didn't know why I did the things I did. They felt like something I couldn't help doing. I think I had expected Dr. Travis to tell me what caused my stuttering and how to stop it and speak normally. What he said was that I was to lie on the couch and keep on talking about anything and everything I most wanted to talk about, and I did that all through the fall and winter and spring.

Finally I got up off the couch and started doing something else with the hope that it would help me speak better. Dr. Travis and his chief in the department of psychiatry, Dr. Samuel T. Orton, were interested in testing out the theory that stuttering is related somehow to handedness. We could find no evidence that I had ever been left-handed. In fact, my good right arm had seen me through many a victory or thrilling defeat on the baseball field and basketball court. In the interests of science, however, and with the unreasoning anticipations of a prospector, I set myself the slightly baffling objective of becoming left-handed. Ten years and countless bruises later, having become a threat to my own thumbs, I placed in storage the many ingenious braces and mittens Dr. Arthur Steindler had helped me design, put away my left-handed scissors, and with my right hand wrote "Finis" to the experiment, still stuttering splendidly.

As it turned out these were only two of the many clinical experiments I was to do on myself and others at Iowa. After two years the university awarded me a bachelor's degree — but I was stuttering about as much as ever. So I stayed. In fact, I moved into the laboratory, no longer just a "guinea pig" but also a graduate student majoring in speech pathology. I had decided to specialize in my own ordeal.

At the end of another year, I was given a master's degree. My problem not yet solved, I continued and there came a day in 1931 when a doctoral degree was conferred upon me. With need and curiosity undiminished, for I was still stuttering, I went on, and then one day the director of the laboratory, Dr. Travis, left — and there I was.

I am like the man who was asked, "How did you come to fall in the lake?" and he said, "I didn't. I came to fish."

◆　◆　◆

It was in 1934 that I became keenly aware that although there were many different opinions about stuttering and its causes, nothing like a planned and thorough scientific study of how the problem begins had ever been made. With a resolution to put first things as nearly first as possible at such a late date, I soon found myself, with several friends and associates at the Iowa Speech Clinic, engaged in a search for the beginnings of the problem called stuttering. What started out as a spirited exercise of curiosity turned into more than a quarter-century of research. This book is the story of that research and of a comprehensive program of related efforts to discover what causes stuttering — in order to find out how to prevent it and to treat it effectively.

How would you have gone about the job of finding out how the problem of stuttering begins? What would you have looked for? Where? What questions would you have put to whom? Why those questions? Why to those persons?

We quickly discovered that there were several decisions we had to make before we could even get our investigation under way. Some of these decisions were surprisingly difficult. Some were easy. It took no great deliberation to decide, first of all, to concentrate on cases in which the problem of stuttering had arisen very recently. The point of this, of course, was to get case histories that were as detailed and reliable as possible. But before we could determine how recently the problem had begun we had to come to grips with an incredibly knotty question: *How could we tell whether or not a child had begun to stutter?*

How would you have answered this question? If you are like most other people, you would probably say, "Why, anybody can tell whether or not a child is stuttering by the way he talks." And yet, how does a child talk if he is stuttering — *for the first time in his life*, that is? Again, if you are like most other people, you would be likely to say that he talks with hesitations and repetitions in his speech. But even normal speakers, at all age levels, speak with hesitations and repetitions, some with few, some with many. You hesitate sometimes in speaking, stumble over sounds, repeat words, and the like. How can you tell by listening to your child, or any other child, whether he is speaking with "too many" hesitations? How many are "too many"? Would you say that a youngster who hesitates and re-

peats more than the average child is a stutterer? If so, then by definition all children who repeat more than "the average child" — and that
means roughly half of all children — are to be classified as stutterers!

If you don't use "the average" as the dividing line, where do you
draw the line between children you regard as stutterers and those you
regard as normal speakers? Do you pick the 5 per cent who are the
most hesitant and repetitious? Or 10 per cent? Or 1 per cent? Can
you make your measurements exact enough to do this? What do you
do about the problem of variation? That is, your child, or any other
youngster, may speak much more smoothly at one time than another,
or in talking to one person than when talking to someone else. Is he,
then, a stutterer part of the time but not all the time? And how are
you to compare your child's speech with that of other youngsters?
Should you, perhaps, compare your child's speech with that of other
children only when they are speaking under the same or similar conditions? Or is it sufficient to compare your youngster's speech with
that of other children on the basis of a general impression gained by
listening to children wherever and whenever you happen to hear
them speaking?

How, indeed, can you tell whether your child, or any child, "has
begun to stutter"?

It was most impressive to discover in 1934 that there was no
clearly satisfactory answer to this utterly fundamental question. It
seemed to us a very serious matter that for years, for centuries in
fact, men had gone ahead to spin theories about stuttering before
they had made quite clear what they were spinning theories about.
After all, it is hardly possible to explain the beginning of something
if we are not able to tell whether or not it has begun. And how is it
possible to prevent or treat something if we cannot explain very well
how it begins — what causes it, that is?

We simply had to find a better answer than had so far been thought
of to the question of how to tell whether or not a child has begun to
stutter. Until we could do this, it was not possible to proceed with
our investigation of how stuttering begins.

After long deliberation, we finally decided that we would accept
as a stutterer, for the purposes of our research, any youngster

brought to us by his parents as a stutterer. We concluded, in other words, that the soundest way to set about finding "new stutterers" was just to let it be known that we were looking for them, and then sit back and see if any children were brought to us. If any were, then we could examine them — and their parents — to find out what they were like. It was no good making up our minds what they would be like before examining them.

As it turned out, we were wiser than we knew at the time, because this decision had the effect of focusing our attention in each case upon *the problem* called "stuttering." We did not understand then as clearly as we did later that the word "stuttering" is, indeed, whatever else it may be, a name for a problem. And, as we came to see more and more clearly, the problem called stuttering includes much more than hesitations and repetitions in speech. It also includes certain feelings and reactions of the listener. That is, the problem called stuttering involves not only a speaker and his way of speaking and his related feelings, but also his listeners and the feelings they have about his way of speaking and the reactions they make to it. It was this total problem on which our attention was focused by the practical decision we made — for the simple reason that whenever a mother and father feel their child is stuttering, *they* at least have a problem. And if the parents continue to have the problem, the child is also likely to be caught up in it sooner or later.

Between 1934 and 1939, when we completed Study I, as we have come to refer to it, forty-six children, thirty-two boys and fourteen girls, were brought to us by their parents, quite soon after the parents had decided they were beginning to stutter. They ranged in age from about two to nine years, and had an average age of slightly over four years. The average interval between onset of the problem, as reported, and our first interview was only about five and one-half months. We followed the development of these children for an average period of two and a half years.

For each child who had been "diagnosed" by his parents as a stutterer, and brought to us for clinical advice and help, we also selected and studied another child of the same age, sex, and level of intelligence, who was thought by his parents to have normal speech.

12

When we first started to investigate these two groups of children, we were not at all sure what we would find. Mainly, we were very curious. We certainly expected to find differences of some sort between the two groups of children. On the basis of theories current in the mid-thirties it was to be expected that more of the children classified as stutterers would have suffered birth injuries and diseases, and more of them would have developed slowly and been awkward or lacking in muscular coordination. It was also to be expected, on the basis of most textbooks then in use, that the children classified as stutterers would be more nervous or emotionally disturbed, insecure, shy, or socially immature than the other youngsters. True, such theories were generally vague, so that it was not clear just what details were supposed to be found, or looked for, in actual cases. The fact is that so little scientific research had been done that the theories were largely unsupported by data, but they were the theories that were then generally taken for granted and our thinking was in some measure affected by them.

As it turned out, what we actually discovered was surprisingly different from what we had expected to find.

◆   ◆   ◆

Before getting into the details of what we found, however, there is a particularly fundamental point to be made as clearly as possible. It has to do with questions and answers. When we began our investigation of how stuttering begins we supposed that the questions we were asking were fairly simple and we were hardly prepared for the great difficulty the mothers and fathers had in nearly every case in giving us a straightforward account of their child's history. If they had more than one child, they seemed not always to be sure which one they were talking about. In discussing the child's birth or medical history they could not always recall what the doctor had told them, and they sometimes seemed unsure of what he had meant by what he had said. The parents often found it difficult, indeed impossible, to pinpoint an event to the particular day, or even week or month or year, of its occurrence. They could not always remember the places where things had happened. They used expressions such as "about average" or "a little slow" or "very good" without appearing to know what these terms might mean so far as children generally are concerned. Usually they seemed to be comparing their child with one or two other children they happened to know, instead of using reliable norms for the general population of children of like age and sex.

After several years of clinical interviewing, I have become highly sensitive to the fact that most persons are apparently not used to speaking with accuracy and in detail about their own experiences or those of their children. Most of us become accustomed to a certain level of vagueness, and evidently it is difficult and even unpleasant for us to try very hard for any length of time to be much less vague, or more careful and clear, then we usually are. An interviewer must try, therefore, to cultivate unusual sympathy and patience, as well as a special skill in asking questions effectively. He learns to sense the difference between an answer that is a clear description and one that is a statement of judgment, or opinion, or prejudice, or sheer imagination. He must finally accept a fundamental limitation on human knowledge: it is impossible to find out everything about anything.

It is as important to know what we don't know, and especially what we can never know, as it is to be clear about what we do know or can manage somehow to find out sometime. Without a sense of the limitations of our possible knowledge (which means, in part, an awareness of our ignorance) we cannot judge very well the value of what we do know and of what we are told by others — who so often manage somehow to sound as though they know what they are talking about.

And so in scores of intensive interviews during the course of our research program I have encouraged mothers and fathers to tell in their own words, as clearly and fully as they could, just what the facts had been in the beginning of the problem they called stuttering, so far as they could recall the facts. I wanted of course to get all the specific details I could. But I also wanted to explore the limits of *obtainable* information. I wanted to find out what it was that the only possible informants — the only observers who were on hand at the moment when the problem first arose — were unable to report. I was intent on determining as best I could what it was that they had forgotten or had not observed in the first place.

The best way I know to make the meaning of these generalities come alive on the printed page is to let you listen in, as it were, on a few clinical interviews. In the next chapter you will be able to see for yourself just what it is that parents are able — and unable — to say when asked to give information about their own youngsters doing specific things that the parents have called "stuttering" in particular situations at specific times. These were actual interviews, tape recorded and transcribed. All names, however, are changed and certain telltale details are disguised.

These tape-recorded materials are printed with permission of the persons concerned. I am tremendously grateful to them. They were cooperative and long-suffering in response to a kind and intensity of questioning that they could have been pardoned for resenting. Their understanding of our unusual purposes — and so of our uncommon procedures — was not merely helpful, it was utterly essential to the success of our research.

CHAPTER 2

Alice and Her Mother

IF YOU feel that your child is stuttering, how well do you think you would be able to answer these two questions: Exactly what was your youngster doing, in what situation, when you first had the idea that he was beginning to stutter? Just when — at what moment of what day — was this?

Could you be more precise than the young father whose answers are transcribed below from a tape-recorded interview?

FATHER (F): As a matter of fact, if you want to pin it down I would say the last three or four weeks is when this that we thought was a speech block — I don't know if that's the term you use . . .

INTERVIEWER (I): That's all right — whatever your word is for it.

F: . . . came into the picture. It's the last three or four weeks that he has started doing this.

I: Umhm. Well, let's get at the very beginnings of this thing that you're talking about now. You say the last three or four weeks. Now, can you be a little more definite? Can you — can you name the day?

F: I couldn't at all.

I: Let's see, this is April 23rd. Do you remember April Fools' Day this year? Did your kids do any monkeyshines that you can remember?

F: Well, now, as I recall, that was also Easter this year.

I: That's right, Easter Sunday.

F: And there were no monkeyshines as far as April Fools' was concerned. Everything was concentrated on Easter.

I: You remember Easter?

F: Yes, I can remember Easter.

I: Did you do something special? Did you go to church?

F: Yes, went to church and washed the car — that was a fairly warm day as I recall, so I know they wore their new clothes.

16

I: Was there a special ceremony at church?

F: Oh yes.

I: Did the children participate in it?

F: One or two of them did, I think, sing in the, uh, program.

I: Did the little boy go along?

F: No. He's too young.

I: Umhm. But can you remember his talking on Easter Sunday?

F: No, not at all.

I: Do you remember though, using Easter as a kind of reference point, whether you had worried about his speech before Easter?

F: I can't recall that we did.

I: No?

F: And come to think of it, that's only three weeks ago, too.

I: That's right. Now, then, has anything happened — did you take a trip after Easter?

F: No.

I: Did you make a speech anywhere? I remember one day you told me you were going to Peoria or some place to make a speech.

F: Well, I've made a number of those since Easter in my work.

I: Do you remember the dates of any of them?

F: Not the exact dates, no, because there have been so many of them.

I: Well, can you remember — sometimes I've been able to pinpoint a thing like this because a father came home from a trip and he noticed for the first time, he thought, that —

F: Well, now, as I recall, I think my wife said, "There goes Billy again. He's — " and then I noticed it.

I: When was this?

F: Now, I don't know. I mean — I mean back in the last week or so.

I: Well, today's Monday. It was last Thursday, wasn't it, you first mentioned this to me that day downtown?

F: Well, I mentioned it last Thursday or Friday.

I: That was April the 19th or 20th then. Now, you can't remember — you said at that time it had been a couple of weeks.

F: Yes, I said it — you know, I used the term very loosely.

I: That would put it back to the fourth or fifth, along in there. Was it, do you remember was it during the middle of the week or was it . . .

F: No.

I: . . . or was it a weekend? Did you have people in?

F: No. No, I don't — the thing is that you're trying to get at some particular date, and dates mean nothing to me here other than just a relative time, I mean — and I say two weeks, and it could have

17

been three weeks, or it could have been a little before Easter, although that seems a little too far back. It's been the last three or four —

We never did succeed in finding out the exact time (and so the situation or incident) that marked "the beginning" of the problem in this case, although the father's memory, and the mother's too in another interview, were being directed back only three or four weeks.

This father and mother are not unusual. We discovered that even the parents of a young child like this one, reporting soon after onset of the problem, do not usually refer to a specific day, hour, or incident, but tend rather to say "Johnny began to stutter when he was three" or "last summer" or, as here, "a few weeks ago." And where the informants are adult stutterers or the parents of older children it is practically impossible to obtain anything like precise information. Likewise the parents we interviewed usually found it difficult to say what they had meant by "stuttering" the first time they used the word in referring to their children's speech.

Yet we simply have to be able to locate the beginning of the problem accurately in place and time, not only in a general sort of way. We need a clear account of the first instance of whatever it was that someone thought of as stuttering. Unless we can get this in a particular case we can only guess what the circumstances actually were, and unless we can obtain this sort of information in many cases we can have no solid foundation for any assertions we may make about the nature of stuttering at its onset and the causes of it. Without this solid foundation we are necessarily on shaky ground in recommending any specific kind of treatment to you or to anyone else concerned with the problem.

Fairly lengthy excerpts from the transcript of a tape-recorded interview with the mother of a five-year-old girl illustrate with unusual clarity the process of patient exploration to be carried out in the attempt to get at the beginnings of the problem, to find out exactly what it was that a particular set of parents called stuttering and precisely when and where they had begun to feel there was a problem.

The parents, whom we shall call the Smiths, had come to the University of Iowa Speech Clinic with the child, and the mother was interviewed at the end of a day of clinical examinations. It was known before starting the interview, therefore, that the little girl's intelligence was superior, that she had a relatively large vocabulary, and that her level of social maturity was a little beyond her age. Even so, she was not very enthusiastic about her first taste of school. She had made a perfect score on a test of her ability to form all the speech sounds, she had normal hearing and good coordination of her speech muscles, and she had talked with rather ordinary ease and fluency at various times during the day to three different speech examiners. It had also been determined that the personalities of the mother and father were within the normal range, as evaluated by means of a widely used personality test, and that apparently neither of them was disturbed emotionally in any clinically significant way.

The parts of the transcript that follow have been edited where necessary to make them more readable and to remove or disguise possibly identifying details. The tones of voice cannot, of course, be captured on the printed page, and the thoughtful pauses, the sudden starts, the slowing down and trailing off of certain remarks, the nearly inaudible wonderings, the smiles and frowns and looks of puzzlement — these must be foregone. The interview was carried on in a leisurely, sympathetic, and searching manner. This kind of intensive interviewing is very demanding of the investigator; certainly most parents feel that it is extremely trying for them. It is essential that the interviewer do his best, therefore, to balance persistence with kindness and considerateness, and in this particular interview such a balance was achieved to at least a generally satisfactory degree.

INTERVIEWER (I): Mrs. Smith, what is your daughter's name?

MRS. SMITH (MS): Alice.

I: And how old is she?

MS: Five.

I: What is the problem?

MS: She has, uh, well, we've been calling it stuttering between ourselves, but it's a repetition of words when she goes to talk.

I: Uh — could you imitate it for me?

MS: I I I I — things like that.

I: Umhm. Has this — uh — had a beginning?

MS: Yes, overnight beginning.

19

I: An overnight beginning? When did it occur?

MS: When she was two and a half.

I: This was, then, in 1953?

MS: That, uh, early that spring or late that winter, I believe.

I: Do you know the date?

MS: No, no I don't.

I: You say that it happened overnight?

MS: It did. I mean I remember the day, but I don't remember the date. She just started.

I: By "overnight" do you mean she woke up in the morning doing it?

MS: One, one morning she came to the kitchen, and, and in a very cute way, as two-and-a-half-year-olds have, began, uh, stuttering that way.

I: First of all, if I can find out a little more about exactly when this happened I'd like to do that. Was it before Easter?

MS: Oh, yes, yes — yes, I'm sure it was before, before that April.

[In this interview the clinician was leading up to an investigation of whatever Alice had done that her mother, or someone, had first regarded as stuttering. Unless this could be spotted precisely in time and place it would not be possible to get a dependable description of the circumstances closely surrounding it. The clinician was quite persistent, therefore, in trying to track down the day, hour, and minute of the onset of the problem. Exact dates seem to be difficult, however, for most of us to recall, except very special ones like anniversaries or those that mark outstanding occurrences. Consequently in interviewing it is sometimes helpful to try to tie one event to another in time — to relate the beginning of the stuttering problem, for example, to "the big flood," or a wedding, or a move to a new home, or the like. The next question asked Mrs. Smith sought such a link].

I: What happened that spring that you can remember? Did anybody get married, or die, or —?

MS: No, sir.

I: There was a flood or a snowstorm?

MS: No, sir, I cannot trace anything at all.

I: A fire or anything else you can remember?

MS: It was an average weekend, an average time — I can think of nothing that could have started it.

I: Well, I'm trying to get some kind of a landmark.

MS: I, I wish we could.

I: Well, anyway, it was perhaps in April.

MS: We'll say before April.

I: Fifteenth of March?

MS: We can — we can say any date. I can't remember exactly.

I: All right. Sometime in March?

MS: All right.

[So often we simply have to settle for something less than the accuracy we would like to achieve. In trying to obtain information, as in other things, we have to learn to get along as well as we can with the best we can do. In this case it turned out that we could do fairly well, because Mrs. Smith was able to relate the apparent beginning of the problem to a specific place and situation, and to the day of the week even though she could not recall the date.]

MS: I would, I would say it was on a, on a Saturday. I remem — (pause) I remember that because Mother and Dad stopped in on the way to whatever they were attending on Friday and Alice was still fine, because we remembered as we traced back she was still fine. Then they returned on Monday unexpectedly going some place and remarked to me that they noticed the change from Friday, and we too had noticed it by Saturday and Sunday.

I: You'd noticed it before your parents pointed it out to you?

MS: Oh, yes.

I: You'd noticed it Saturday?

MS: Yes sir, I, I seem to — (pause)

I: Friday night there had been nothing at all wrong?

MS: Nothing at all wrong.

I: Now then, taking that particular Friday night as our point of reference, tell me how her speech had been before that.

MS: Well, she was just two and a half and was uh, how do they speak — their small sentences — and, and just fine, just as normal as our other child.

I: Well, could you try to tell me about it, about *her* speech rather than the speech of other two-year-olds? And, by the way, can you personally remember what you are telling me? Are you talking from a vivid and specific memory?

MS: I can — may I say this — I can only remember that I found nothing different in her speech from the youngster who was born the year before.

I: Not knowing what her speech was like, the youngster born the year before, I don't quite know, of course, what you are telling me.

21

MS: I see. Well I would say she spoke very normally.

[In talking about the past we tend to repeat general accounts, or family legends, rather than to describe clear visual or auditory memories of specific scenes. It is not that a clear, discrete remembrance is necessarily to be trusted with respect to its accuracy, but it is important to determine whether the informant is talking out of a vivid personal "picture in the head" or is speaking without reference to any particular scene in a given place at a specific hour of an indicated day. We also take for granted that others would use the same words we would and mean the same things by them. Most of the people we talk to, of course, don't need to know exactly what we mean in the way that a doctor or a speech clinician does. It is possible, therefore, that Mrs. Smith had never before been asked a question quite like the next one that was put to her, and it is not to be wondered at that she didn't find it very easy to answer.]

I: What do you mean by "normally"?

MS: Sentences and uh, well I was proud of her. I thought she was doing very well. (Thoughtful pause.) I may not be answering you very well, sir. I'm sorry.

I: Well, that's all right. You just answer the best you can. I may not be asking you very well. Uh — I'm also doing the best I can. It's very difficult to get or to give this kind of information.

MS: I wish we had come sooner. I would remember maybe better.

I: Perhaps. It hasn't been long though, two and a half years.

MS: It seems long.

I: Yes. (Pause.) What, what did you expect of her speech at the age of two?

MS: What did I expect? No sir, I, I don't know exactly how to answer that. Everything went along — (pause)

I: All right?

MS: I did not expect her to stutter.

[If there is one point to be stressed more than any other in explaining the problem of finding out how stuttering begins, it is that most parents take for granted that "stuttering" has a standard meaning. They use the word as though it served to *describe* rather than to *classify* what the speaker does. If, for example, you tell me your child stutters, and the next day someone asks me to describe what your child does I would have to say that I didn't know. You would only have told me that you had classified what he does as "stuttering" but you would not have described what you had classified. It seemed necessary, therefore, to try at this point to help Mrs. Smith recall just what it was that Alice had done.]

I: I don't know what, what you mean by the word "stutter."

MS: That's right. I use that term — (voice trailed off)

I: What is it you didn't expect her to do? How would you say it without using the word "stutter"?

MS: I see. I did not expect her to, uh, have difficulty in saying —

I: It would help if you were to say it in some more descriptive way than "have difficulty." What did she do that you did not expect?

MS: Keep repeating her, uh, the word.

I: Keep repeating?

MS: Such as I I I I want to guh guh guh go — like that, you see.

I: I see. You didn't expect her to do this at the age of two?

MS: Well, I, I — no, I was surprised when she did.

I: I see. You felt, then, that she had never done that before this particular Friday night?

MS: No, she hadn't, that's right. Before this particular Saturday morning she had never done that.

[The interviewer was trying at this point to determine, so far as this was possible, whether Mrs. Smith was making statements about Alice's speech or about herself, her personal memories of Alice's speech, her habits of listening to Alice when Alice was very young. Since the interviewer knew, as a result of completed studies of the speech of young children, that probably no child speaks without doing a certain amount of repeating and hesitating, he was tuned particularly to Mrs. Smith's statements that Alice had never done anything like that. The most likely interpretation to be placed on her statements to this effect was that she had never noticed Alice's hesitations and repetitions before the Saturday in question. If that was, in fact, the case, then why had she begun to notice them on that particular Saturday? Did Alice speak with more or longer repetitions than ever before on that day? Or was Mrs. Smith more attentive to such things that morning? Or was there something else in the situation? The investigator's questions were designed to clarify these aspects of the picture. What follows, as a result of the further questioning, is one of the clearest descriptions we have ever been able to obtain of what seems to have been the very first instance of a child's speech that a parent had classified as "stuttering."]

I: Uh, then I want to know a little more about what it was she did that Saturday morning that she had never done before. Can you tell me quite exactly what that was like? Now, you have already tried to, but please try again.

MS: I seem to remember working in the kitchen and Alice walking in from playing with her older sister.

I: How old was her older sister?

MS: Seventeen months older.

I: Umhm.

MS: They came in from the living room and Alice began telling me something and said, "I I I I," the way I told you before.

I: Can you remember the exact word that she said?

MS: It was "I" — the first word I ever noticed.

I: What was the rest of the sentence?

MS: I don't recall. (Pause.) I don't recall.

I: Do you recall whether she finished the sentence?

MS: Yes, she finished the sentence.

I: Then, do you recall at least in a vague way whether it was a long or a short sentence?

MS: It was a short sentence, I would say.

I: And did she repeat any other words in it?

MS: Not then.

I: Just the "I" with which it began?

MS: Yes, sir.

I: How many times did she repeat the "I"?

MS: Maybe like three or four.

I: Three or four. Now, how confident would you say we could be of this answer?

MS: Well, I'd feel sure, sir, it was no more than that.

I: No more? Might it have been less? Two or three?

MS: Maybe two or three. Two to four.

I: Two to four? All right. Was the word "I" repeated from two to four times with a great, uh, show of effort? Or was it done rather lightly or almost casually?

MS: I would say it was almost casually.

I: Almost casually? Umhm. Did Alice seem to be highly aware of it?

MS: No. I would say — (pause)

24

I: Was she aware of it at all as far as you could tell?

MS: Then? No.

I: No. All right. So then one Saturday morning you noticed that she said "I" two to four times without tension, without her being apparently aware that she was doing it. And then she went ahead and she spoke the rest of the words in the sentence all right?

MS: Yes.

I: And this is what you have regarded, is it, as the beginning of what you call her "stuttering"?

MS: Yes, sir.

[This is, indeed, an unusually clear account of the beginning of the problem. In very few cases is it possible to get a description of the first instance of that which someone has taken to be stuttering. Mrs. Smith's account, moreover, appeared to be consistent with the general conclusion drawn from our research on the onset of stuttering that in most cases the hesitations and repetitions first regarded as "stuttering" are usually not very remarkable. What Mrs. Smith was describing seemed to be the sort of thing the average youngster does roughly 50 times every 1,000 running words. In this basic sense, then, it was apparently a normal type of speech disfluency that she was describing. If that was true, the major question to be answered was, not why had Alice begun to repeat words or sounds, but why had Alice's mother begun to notice that she was doing that sort of thing, and why was she concerned about it? The interviewer tried to obtain as much detail as he possibly could that would be relevant to these questions.]

I: I want to take this inch by inch as it were. Now, what happened immediately after what we have just talked about? She said, "I I I I," or something like that and finished the sentence. Who spoke next?

MS: I answered her probably.

I: What did you say? Do you know? You may not know the answers to some of these questions, of course.

MS: No. I merely answered or explained whatever she was, whatever she wanted, wanted to know.

I: You don't know what this was?

MS: No, but I made no reference to her manner of asking me.

I: Do you remember exchanging glances with the sister?

MS: No.

25

I: Did the sister seem to notice it?

MS: Not then. Not that particular time.

[Even though Mrs. Smith was very cooperative, she had a certain amount of difficulty following the interviewer's line of inquiry in this close questioning. He was trying to trace the beginnings of the problem minute by minute. It is not often that one has an opportunity to obtain an account as detailed as this one was proving to be. He wanted, therefore, to get all the facts he could, and to explore the limits beyond which no information could be obtained. Mrs. Smith, not accustomed, naturally, to thinking in terms of such precise recollection, seemed to take for granted that he was asking general instead of extremely precise questions. He was intent on piecing out that specific Saturday minute by minute, or at least as exactly as might prove feasible, but as the following part of the interview indicates, it is nearly impossible to recapture even a day, to say nothing of an hour or a moment, from out of the past.]

I: I want to know what happened next. I want to get this down in a sequence.

MS: Yes, sir, but I don't recall — I don't recall another thing on that day.

I: Can you remember whether the little girl walked back into the living room after you answered her?

MS: Probably she did, but I can't say exactly.

I: What you do remember, then, is that for the rest of that day you did not pay any attention to Alice's speech?

MS: No, sir.

I: There was nothing about it that attracted your attention that day?

MS: This continued from that time on.

I: Pardon me, I don't follow.

MS: Her speech — the way she began talking.

I: From that time on?

MS: From that time on it has continued —

I: On this day? Let's stay with this day. This Saturday. Incidentally, what time of the morning did this happen, what you told me?

MS: Uh, mid-morning, I would say.

I: All right. Now, from then till noon was there anything that you noticed?

MS: No, sir.

I: From noon until time for dinner? That day.

MS: Pardon me — do you mean did I notice her speaking that way again?

I: Yes.

MS: Yes, sir, she continued speaking that way.

I: What did you mean a while ago? I'm not quite sure I follow you. What did you mean a while ago when you said you didn't notice anything the rest of the day?

MS: I thought you were searching for an incident that perhaps could have occurred and I, I can say nothing about that.

I: Well, what is it, then, that you are talking about when you say that she continued that day?

MS: She continued hesitating when she spoke.

I: You call this "hesitating" now. It's the same thing?

MS: Well, I don't know what to call it. I wish someone would give me a word.

I: No, you did, I thought, perfectly well a while ago when you spoke of it as repetition.

MS: Yes, all right. I'll stick to that. That's the same thing.

I: Is that exactly what happened?

MS: Repetition of words, that's right. I'll call it that.

I: All right. Now this you say she did some more of that day?

MS: Yes, sir.

I: But you can't remember specific instances of it?

MS: No, sir, I can't recall any.

I: So, you're not talking out of a specific memory of how you heard her at some specific moment that day any time after mid-morning?

MS: I know that every time she spoke she spoke with repetition of words from then on.

I: You say *every* time she spoke?

MS: Oh, yes, sir. I can't quote what she said, but I know that it occurred again and again.

[The language of every day is marked by common expressions which serve most of our ordinary needs fairly well, but are too lacking in accuracy for certain of our special purposes. Some of these common expressions, such as "I've told him a million times" or "He got red as a beet," are exaggerations. The words "always" and "never" are exaggerations in many of their uses; someone once said that "always" and "never" are two words one should always remember never to use! We form habits of using such words and expressions without stopping to consider whether they say precisely what we mean. With

27

such considerations in mind, the interviewer continued talking with Mrs. Smith.]

I: Has she up to today — every time she has spoken — has she done this, up to today?

MS: She has spells now where she does very well and then — (pause)

I: So it isn't every time she's spoken since that morning?

MS: No, sir.

I: But that day it was every time?

MS: Well — (sigh, long thoughtful pause). I see more clearly what you mean whether — uh, I can't be positive. I'm sorry, Doctor.

I: I see.

MS: I can't be positive whether every time she talked it occurred that day. I'll change that then. I won't say *every* time.

I: All right. What will you say, instead of that?

MS: I noticed it — I continued to notice it occurring when she spoke, but I can't say that it was *every* time she said something. Maybe on certain words.

I: Might it have been once more that day?

MS: Oh, I would say several times more, because children do a lot of talking in a day's time.

I: Twenty times more perhaps?

MS: (Long pause.)

I: What I'm trying to get at is — was this a great, sudden, tremendous outburst of this sort of thing, or did you have your attention called to it this particular Saturday morning, and then a few more times during the day you noticed something like this? Or were you simply appalled by a tremendous display?

MS: No, sir. I, as I said, at first I found it cute, but then — and I thought well, in a few days — a little while — it'd be all over. And I gave it — I tried to give it no thought as to worry.

I: But this was something — something *not* to worry about?

MS: I didn't think it was anything to worry about when it happened. No, sir.

[One of the most interesting and, I think, important things parents do in such interviews as this is to say, as Mrs. Smith did essentially in the remark just quoted, that "at first they were not worried," or "it didn't seem to be anything serious," or "it seemed cute at first." Such statements usually fit with the account given — when one can be given — of what the child was doing when the parents first got the idea that he was "stuttering." As Mrs. Smith described what Alice had done, it does seem that it should not have caused anyone to worry. Nevertheless, in this as in other cases, what the child was doing "at first" was not disregarded. The line between "noticing" something and "worrying" about it is often dim and hard to find. One of the most important purposes of our research has been to find out as much as possible about the course of events that leads from unremarkable sorts of behavior, such as Alice Smith's "I I I I" and her mother's noticing it but not worrying about it, to the serious problems that so often develop from these seemingly unlikely beginnings. And so in talking with Mrs. Smith the interviewer pursued this aspect of the puzzle.]

I: You did not worry about what Alice did that Saturday morning — but you noticed it? It somehow arrested your attention?

MS: I did notice it and others seemed to notice it.

I: Why did you notice it that first Saturday morning? As I recall, you said Alice's older sister did not seem to notice it. The others, by the way, that you say also noticed it did not observe it that first Saturday morning, I assume, because they weren't there.

MS: They weren't there — (thoughtful pause)

I: Let's stay on this particular Saturday for a while longer.

MS: Yes, sir.

I: I want to be very thorough. I want to know exactly what happened when it started, because I want to find out if I can why you noticed it. What did you think there was strange about what Alice did?

MS: Well, I noticed it — I noticed it because it seemed strange to me that she should repeat her word that way. She had never done so before.

I: Now tell me just a little bit about the older girl's speech. Has it been all right?

MS: Yes, sir.

I: Did she ever repeat words?

MS: Not that I noticed, sir.

I: You didn't notice?

MS: I never noticed. Now, I've read, too, that all children do it, but I have never noticed it with Ruth.

[It was beginning to seem clear that Mrs. Smith had not previously been tuned in, so to speak, to the repetitions and hesitations in the speech of her children. For some reason, however, she did pay attention to the repeating that Alice did on the particular Saturday in question. While it is not certain that the repeating Alice did that day was out of the ordinary, nevertheless one way to proceed with the investigation that might bring more facts to light was to assume that Alice had been doing something that needed to be accounted for.]

I: Now, then, let's take all this at face value, and try to account for it. What is your theory? Why do you think this happened on that particular day?

MS: I have — I do not know why it happened that day —

I: Well, this is of special interest to me, and I want to find out all I can about what did happen, you see, just before or at the time . . .

MS: I wish I knew.

I: If *nothing* happened, this is a rather important fact. Alice had not been sick?

MS: No, sir.

I: She had not been in any accident?

MS: No, sir.

I: There's one theory of stuttering which relates it to handedness. Was she using the right hand or the left hand?

MS: She was using her right hand.

I: She always had as far as you know?

MS: As far as I — I handed things to her right hand when she began learning to eat. I have seen her use her left hand. I think all small children do.

I: I see. You think that she might have had some difficulty about her handedness at this time?

MS: No, sir.

I: Not that you know of?

MS: No, sir.

[Mrs. Smith's reaction to this line of questioning, as shown especially in her next response, was of some significance. She was beginning to wonder why she noticed Alice's speech when she did. This was, of course, the basic question to be answered. Moreover, she seemed to be indicating quite clearly that, although she had undoubtedly been convinced that Alice had begun to stutter that Saturday morning, she had not been greatly impressed with the seriousness of whatever it was that Alice had done. This would seem to be added evidence that she had not done very much. It was important, therefore, to achieve as much clarification of this matter as seemed possible.]

I: Now, uh, she had not been somehow frightened?

MS: No, sir. And all this did not seem very important to me at the time. Perhaps that's why I can't remember the details as I should. It didn't seem important. I wish I could. (Pause.) I wonder why I noticed what I noticed that weekend? I wonder why?

I: That morning when she came in the kitchen, had she done this several times or was this the first you had seen of her that morning?

MS: That's the first — no, no, I had seen her that morning. That's the first time I noticed it.

I: She had been at breakfast?

MS: I had dressed her, fed her, and she was playing.

I: She had talked in her usual way?

MS: Yes, sir.

I: Her usual fine way, nothing wrong?

MS: I didn't notice anything, sir. I didn't notice this.

I: All right.

MS: I don't know why I started to — (thoughtful pause)

I: All right. So then, suddenly in the middle of the morning after she had been talking up to that hour of that day so that you had not noticed anything . . .

MS: I had not —

I: . . . then all of a sudden in the middle of the morning of this day you noticed something?

MS: Yes, sir.

[The interviewer now returns to a very important consideration. Nearly all the parents in our studies of the onset of stuttering have said that before their children had, as they put it, begun to stutter by repeating sounds and words, or hesitating in other ways, they had never done such things. Our parents must actually have meant that until the child's speech and language development had proceeded to a certain point, they had not paid any attention to the fluency, or disfluency, of his speaking. If that is true, then when a child's parents finally begin to give attention to his disfluencies they are likely to be more or less surprised by the number of them, and so might very well conclude that something is wrong — and that what is wrong is something new, when they are actually referring to something the child has been doing all along. The interviewer touched on this aspect of the matter at this point.]

I: And you would have heard — if she were an average child — something like fifty instances of repetition every thousand words. Now, if you'd never noticed it before this might sound like a tremendous lot of trouble — if you were calling it trouble. But if she is like other children she had been doing it the day before and the day before that — about fifty times per thousand words, if she's an average child.

MS: I see. Yes, sir.

I: But now, if you noticed it at all you'd have had that much of it to notice.

MS: Yes, sir, I see what you mean.

I: So, would this have startled you? Would this have —

MS: It amused me. It did not startle me.

I: It amused you at first, but when did it start to worry you?

MS: Oh, I guess it took a month or two months, or —

I: Oh.

MS: I can't, now, I can't describe the day that it actually started worrying me.

I: I see.

[It seems to be reasonably clear that the Smiths had not been particularly concerned about whatever it was that Alice was doing in her speech that weekend. Evidently they did not start worrying about the way she was talking until some months later. As the interview proceeded, Mrs. Smith told of a brief, apparently rather casual conversation she had had with her husband about Alice's speech Saturday evening. A few remarks had also passed between Mrs. Smith and her parents when they stopped by the following Monday.]

I: When was the next time that this was a topic of conversation?

MS: I can't tell you that. I, I can't tell you that. As I say, I didn't become concerned for quite a while.

I: Did you call it stuttering when it first — that Saturday morning?

MS: No, sir.

I: What did you call it — to yourself, that is?

MS: To myself? (Pause.) I don't know. I guess I, I guess I did. I was amused by it. I, I didn't label it — I don't think that I even labeled it though in my mind. It was just that what she did was cute, and, and remained that way for a while.

I: There came a time when you started calling it stuttering — at least to yourself?

MS: To myself? Yes, sir.

[It will be recalled, in relation to these apparently somewhat uncertain and unclear statements of Mrs. Smith, that near the beginning of the interview she had definitely identified the "I I I I" incident as the first instance of what she had meant by "stuttering." The interviewer continued at this point to try to find, if possible, some clue that would explain why Mrs. Smith had been tuned to notice the fluency aspects of Alice's speech, evidently for the first time, on that particular Saturday morning.]

I: Had you ever known any other stutterers?

MS: No, sir.

I: Never known one? In your own family?

MS: None in the family, no, sir. I had a neighbor once who did. A different type, though, I believe.

I: Had this impressed you greatly?

MS: Uh, it was since I was married. I often wanted to, to help her when she would get a period like that.

I: Hmhm.

MS: She would stop — (pause)

I: Had you read anything about stuttering before this Saturday morning.

MS: No, sir. Uh, later on we read in the newspaper about your clinic. I'm sure it was — (pause)

I: How much later?

MS: It was a Sunday paper section.

I: About that time, I mean?

MS: No, sir. It was much later.

I: I see.

MS: I believe the article left me with the impression that I was to ignore it, and it quoted how often all normal children between the ages of two and five repeat — which you told me earlier —

I: I see.

MS: I believe I read that in the article.

I: I see. Well, I believe we'd better call that the end of our interview.

MS: Thank you, Doctor.

I: Well, thank you very much, Mrs. Smith.

◄   ◄   ◄

These interview passages serve to point up certain important features of the problem called stuttering. Although Mrs. Smith's words suggest that her little girl started one day to speak in a new and different way, which she felt was "not right," her account makes quite clear that she had not been alarmed. She indicated, indeed, that she had been more or less amused. Mr. Smith also, according to the mother, took the matter casually. Their only discussion of it at the time had evidently consisted of a brief exchange of incidental remarks. The mother's report indicates that in general the events of the weekend when the little girl "began to stutter" were not important enough to them to be remembered clearly. Mrs. Smith said she had thought that the repeating the little girl was doing was cute, and even though her words (revised later in the interview) were that the child had continued to do it from that time on "every time she spoke," neither she nor the father had considered it a problem to worry about until after two or three months had passed. As time went on, however, the Smiths had done considerable worrying. For example, they had taken Alice to a speech clinic once a week for a few months. Feeling a need for more help, they had eventually arranged to bring Alice to Iowa City.

This pattern — the combination of a few statements that seem to indicate that a grave change in the child's speech had occurred in mid-morning of a particular day, along with a general account of essential disregard of this change (no inclination apparently to call a doctor, get other help, have the child rest, or even discuss the matter) — is characteristic of most of the case histories we have obtained by means of very thorough interviewing of parents soon after reported onset of the problem. The most acceptable implication would seem to be that actually there had been little, if any, significant change in the child's speech, but that rather the parents had begun to notice something that the youngster had been doing before. If there was a change in the child's manner of talking — and it is possible that Alice, for instance, repeated more over the specially remembered weekend than she had previously — it probably occurred in response to a passing upset of some sort, or was, in any case, slight and not something that would be likely to cause much concern for most parents, or for any parents, including the Smiths, unless they are particularly attentive to things such as this that they usually disregard.

Mrs. Smith's account would seem to indicate that once she got the

34

idea that Alice was stuttering, she noticed somewhat more than she had before the repetitions and hesitations in Alice's speech, but not apparently in the speech of other children. In some of our laboratory studies we have seen striking evidence of the way a listener's perception is influenced by the fact that he has already taken for granted that a speaker is a stutterer. In a study by one of my students, Dr. Curtis Tuthill, now a professor of psychology in Georgetown University, several groups of persons were instructed to listen to recordings of speech and to mark on a mimeographed sheet each stuttered word. This instruction implied, of course, that the speakers were stutterers. Actually some parts of the recordings contained samples of the speech of normal speakers, but three out of four of the listeners, with their attention tuned for stuttering, marked some words as stuttered in the normal speech samples. These samples did, of course, contain the usual number of normal or ordinary hemmings and hawings, pauses, repeated words, and the like. Just so, the everyday speech of toddlers is marked by many hesitations and repetitions, and a parent who is listening for "stuttering" tends to hear "it," to notice, that is, the repetitions and to assume that the repetitions are "stuttering."

Once we have decided that a child stutters — or that he is awkward, or exceptionally intelligent, or mentally retarded, or nervous — we are likely to take for granted, within limits, that whatever he does he is stuttering, or being awkward, or sharp, or dull, or nervous. We don't as a rule think of comparing his speech, or other behavior, in a scientifically careful way with that of "most other children" or "the average child" of his age and circumstances. And we do not usually take into account as fully as we should the conditions to which he is reacting at any given time.

The Chinese have a delightfully droll proverb that points up these basic considerations: Get yourself a reputation as an early riser and you can sleep all day.

◀   ◀   ◀

Mrs. Smith's account of Alice's speech behavior is to be read with due appreciation of the fact that it is necessarily expressive of her

35

own feelings and judgments and of the ways of her own distinctive memory. And this is true of any parent's similar account, your own included, or mine. We always talk, in part at least, about ourselves — our own ways of looking and evaluating and feeling, of recalling and forgetting and distorting, and of putting the world about us "into words" — whenever we talk about anything at all. Just as you or I would, so Mrs. Smith revealed the expectations and preconceptions she had had concerning her daughter's speech. Although she said she had read about the hesitations and repetitions to be found normally in the speech of young children, apparently it had not occurred to her to use the information in making a realistic appraisal of the fluency of her own child's speech. In this, Mrs. Smith is typical of many, possibly most, of us. We do not always do very well in applying the knowledge we have about children in general in judging our own youngsters.

This kind of interviewing reveals that nearly all memories are in varying degrees short-term, fragmentary, blurred, and confused. Even so, they are the source of practically the only information we are ever going to get in specific cases about the onset of the problem called stuttering. This can only mean that our data can never be completely or absolutely dependable. We must work harder than we otherwise would, therefore, to determine what the facts are, or may have been, in each case — and then speak with a realization that we cannot possibly know completely what we are talking about. This need not keep us from having convictions, based on the best information we can get, such as it may be. It need only keep us from being unduly dogmatic and from hanging on to old convictions when our best information will not support them.

◀ ◀ ◀

These, then, are some of the thoughts that can be helpful to us as we try to learn all we can about the problem called stuttering. If, as a parent, you have a need to understand this problem, and to do something about it, it is particularly important to bear in mind that alertness begins at home. For the sake of your child it is essential that you recall the facts surrounding the onset of the problem as fully and as accurately as you can. It is equally important that you admit, and reckon with, all that you have forgotten or never knew in the first place.

It is by allowing for our limitations sensibly and wisely that we can make the most effective use of what we have been able to find out about the problem called stuttering. It has been, after all, a very great deal. It has been enough to give direction to the further research from which ever greater benefits can be expected. It has been enough, moreover, to make possible increasingly effective ways of dealing with the problem. With each passing year clinical services are being improved. In the world of all of us who are concerned with the problem called stuttering, the old days were not as good as our new days are certain to be.

CHAPTER 3

Forty-six Unexpected Answers

WE'VE got a bit ahead of ourselves in the chronological story of our research adventure, for by the time of the interview reported in the preceding chapter the interviewer had learned enough not to be surprised at some of the things Mrs. Smith was saying, or not saying — and surprised he surely would have been in the mid-thirties. At that time he would have assumed that any parent bringing a child to a speech clinic as a stutterer would say that one day the youngster had started to hesitate a great deal, or do an excessive amount of repeating, to block in speaking, and to strain. Taking this for granted, the interviewer would have searched for some physical breakdown or perhaps an emotional disturbance of some sort to account for the sudden and distressing breakdown in the child's speech. Study I, then, our first investigation, proved to be a revelation of how very great the difference can be sometimes between what we have come to take for granted and what we find when we look searchingly for facts.

In Study I, and in each of our other investigations of the beginnings of stuttering, we examined a group of children who were brought to a speech clinic as stutterers. We called these children the clinical group. We also studied a like number of children whose parents thought of them as normal speakers, or nonstutterers. We called these the control group. Now, it is to be noted with special thoughtfulness that the word "stutterer" means "a child *classified by some-one* as a stutterer," and the word "nonstutterer" means "a child *classified by someone* as a nonstutterer." The fact that the children had been classified in these different ways by someone, usually their parents, is not, in itself, evidence that the two groups of children were, in fact, different in any way. Whether they actually differed, and if so how, was to be decided on the basis of our research findings, which we shall now review.

◄   ◄   ◄

To consider what might seem to be first things first, the children in Study I had apparently suffered no serious birth injuries, with two possible exceptions. There were eight, two stutterers and six non-stutterers, out of the ninety-two in both groups who underwent some sort of unusual birth conditions that were evidently not serious. For two stutterers birth had been a considerable ordeal. For the less remarkable of these the use of forceps resulted in a mark on the temple which cleared in about four weeks, there was some paralysis of one side of the face for a few hours, and it had proved a bit difficult to get the infant to start breathing. In the more notable case there was a breech delivery and forceps were used; there was some injury to the infant's neck and mouth, as well as to one arm and shoulder; breathing was hard to initiate, pulse was slow at first, and it was difficult to get the baby to start nursing; as the child developed he exhibited some degree of spastic tension. This particular child, however, the only one whose birth injuries were unquestionably grave, was no longer thought of by his parents, or by anyone else, as a stutterer by the end of our study.

For all of the other forty nonstutterers and forty-two stutterers birth was normal according to the best information we could obtain. The relative lack of difference between the two groups of children in this respect was not what we had expected to find.

◄   ◄   ◄

It was also somewhat contrary to expectations that the children classified as stutterers had not shown a slower rate of development than had those in the control group. The average ages at which the children crawled, stood up alone, walked, sat up, got their first teeth, fed themselves, dressed themselves, and said their first words and sentences were essentially the same for both groups. Moreover, both groups were well within the normal range for children generally in these respects.

So it went also for diseases and injuries. In only four cases was any kind of illness possibly related in time to the onset of the stuttering problem. Of these, one child was reported to have had infected tonsils at the time he was first thought to stutter; another was said to have had a cold and sore throat; it was said of the third that he may have been weakened somewhat by pneumonia shortly before he was first regarded as a stutterer; and the fourth child had "very mild measles" at about the time it was felt that he was beginning to stutter. In none of these cases, however, was the illness or its effects serious, and in none was there a clear physical relationship between the illness and the onset of the problem called stuttering. For the other forty-two classified as stutterers, no such relationship was in any way suggested.

Injuries of one sort or another were reported for four of the nonstuttering children and six of those in the clinical group. None of them had any serious aftereffects, and for our purposes there is no need to describe those experienced by the nonstutterers. Of the six stutterers, one was said to have fallen in a bathtub in such a way as to drive a tooth into the upper front gum ridge, but this occurred four months before he was said to have begun to stutter. A minor scalp wound that resulted from an automobile collision occurred nine months before the reported onset of stuttering in another case. In a third case a broken left collarbone, which had healed satisfactorily, preceded the reported onset of stuttering by about one year. Another child had broken his right arm shortly after he was thought to have begun to stutter, and the parents said they had paid close attention in order to see whether his speech was influenced — because they had heard that stuttering might be affected by a change of handedness, and their child had not been able to use his right arm and hand for a time. So far as they could tell the child's speech was neither better nor worse after the accident. In a fifth case the right arm was broken over four years after stuttering had begun; again no effect on the child's speech was observed by the parents while the arm was disabled. The sixth child of this group had merely had a fall which resulted in a minor bruise. In none of these cases did the injury appear to have anything to do with the beginnings of the speech problem.

◀ ◀ ◀

As has been implied, one of the theories current at the time of Study I was that stuttering is caused by changing a left-handed child to right-handedness. It was also supposed by some authorities that more stutterers than nonstutterers are either left-handed or ambidextrous. As a matter of fact, this theory had been given its major support by the Iowa Speech Clinic in the twenties and thirties. We tried to be especially thorough, therefore, in questioning the parents about the handedness of their children and in observing the children themselves.

One of the most important things we had learned from several laboratory studies was that the terms "right-handed," "left-handed," "ambidextrous," "originally right-handed," "originally left-handed," and "changed handedness" were used in very different ways by different people—even by different clinicians and research workers. Also, scores earned on handedness tests by the same individual were found to vary considerably from one kind of test to another.

The basic fact is that normally each of us has two good hands, not just one. When we say that a person is right-handed, for example, we mean that he prefers to use the right hand whenever he has to use one or the other, but we do not mean that he is absolutely unable to use his left hand or that the two hands are in some physical way profoundly different. Most right-handed persons can, if necessary, learn to write and do other things also with the left hand, just as most left-handed persons can, if need be, get along quite well using the right hand.

Using the information we obtained in our study, we judged that thirty-six children in each group were properly classified as right-handed, six stutterers and four nonstutterers as left-handed, and four stutterers and six nonstutterers as ambidextrous.

Twelve of the children classified as stutterers and fourteen of those classified as nonstutterers were judged to have undergone some change in handedness. This was the first study in which anyone had tried to gauge the extent of change of handedness. It was our considered judgment that of the twelve stuttering children who had changed handedness in some degree, two had changed from left to right, two from left to ambidextrous, and eight from ambidextrous to right. Of the fourteen nonstutterers who had changed handedness, one had changed from left to right, two from left to ambidextrous, and eleven from ambidextrous to right. It is of particular interest that full changes from left-handedness to right-handedness were reported for only three of the ninety-two children.

In the mid-thirties all this was news. In fact, there were many to whom these data were simply unbelievable. I was by no means ready to accept the findings myself. Professor Lee Edward Travis, then director of the Iowa Speech Clinic, had done more than anyone else to develop the so-called handedness theory of stuttering. As one of his students, I had been strongly influenced by it. Indeed, as I have recounted in Chapter 1, I tried for ten years to make myself left-handed, and in this effort I was prompted almost wholly by the Travis theory. It was a theory which not only had considerable scholarly authority behind it in those days, but was also in line with popular ways of thinking. That is, it placed the blame for stuttering on a physical condition. Through recorded time most people have leaned toward the view that any really basic explanations of human behavior must be made in terms of muscles, glands, chemistry, and nerve-cells. To most of us anything "psychological" or "environmental" is really pretty hard to grasp.

The so-called handedness theory of stuttering was suggested by the anatomical fact that there are two sides of the brain, and that nerves run from the right side of the brain to the left hand and in general the left side of the body, and from the left side of the brain to the right hand and in general the right side of the body. The speculative part of the theory postulated that in the nonstutterer one side of the brain is somehow "dominant over the other" and controls the discharge of nerve impulses from both sides of the brain so that the two sides of the body receive the same kinds of impulses at the same time. This resulted, it was said, in the coordinated action of the muscles in normal speech. It was assumed that in stutterers neither side of the brain is dominant over the other, so that the two sides act independently of one another, with the result that at any particular instant the two sides of the body may receive different kinds of nerve impulses. This was supposed to account for the action of the speech muscles during stuttering.

It may not be generally recognized, incidentally, that what was referred to as "the dominance of one side of the brain over the other" was never described — because no one ever directly observed any such thing. It was an assumption, or guess, about what might be true. We do not have a standard definition of either "brain dominance" or "handedness." There is no way to be sure, therefore, that "handedness" is related to whatever anyone might intend to convey by "the dominance of one side of the brain over the other," in the absence of clear specification of what is meant by both terms.

One of the more serious difficulties with this theory is that in the kinds of speech reactions called stuttering there is not always muscular incoordination. In fact, Dr. Dean Williams found in a particularly thorough laboratory study at Iowa that the basic coordination of the jaw muscles was the same for both stutterers and nonstutterers. He also found that the things stutterers did when they were said to be stuttering could be generally duplicated by normal speakers. The fine measurements made by Dr. Williams revealed that the coordination between the right and left jaw muscles is not always very good during normal speech, and that the coordination between the two sets of jaw muscles is sometimes very good indeed during stuttering. Moreover, when the stutterers in his study followed instructions to "do their stuttering" in the form of simple repetition of sounds, li li like this, the action of their jaw muscles was the same at it was during their own normal speech — and the same as that of nonstutterers during their speech.

In our first study of the onset of stuttering, in the thirties, we not only obtained information about the handedness of the children but we also made a recommendation about the handedness of each child regarded as a stutterer. We advised that thirty-one of the forty-six so-called stuttering children be consistently right-handed and fifteen left-handed. These recommendations required nine of the children to shift their handedness either from right or ambidexterity to left. The other thirty-seven continued to use the hand they were already using. At the end of the study it did not seem that there had been any relationship between handedness, or recommendations regarding handedness, and the course of improvement or the lack of improvement in the speech of these children.

◀ ◀ ◀

The most important findings of Study I had to do with the problem of stuttering itself — the age at which it was said to have begun, the ways in which the children were speaking when their parents first decided they were stuttering, and how the problem developed after it had arisen.

In half the cases the onset of the problem was said to have occurred between the ages of two years, six months and three years, two months. Why just at that age period? At the time we had no clear answer to this question. The more we thought about it the more remarkable it seemed — but it seemed even more remarkable that such a basic fact had not been well established before.

Indeed, one may never cease marveling at the many facts, quite easy to observe once they are pointed out by someone, that are in our time of the world being observed for the first time. You would think that one of these days we would be done with discovering the obvious! And what really makes a philosopher out of anyone who is thoughtful is the disturbing realization that before we find out the facts about anything we talk confidently and comfortably as though we knew what they were. All too commonly, we do not seem to know that we don't know what we are talking about.

In the matter of the age at which the problem called stuttering arises, we began after much puzzlement and reflection to make sense out of our findings. There does, indeed, seem to be a good reason why a child is more likely to be thought of by his parents as a stutterer when he is around three years old than at any other time. We will go into this more fully later when we come to some of the data we had not yet discovered in the mid-thirties, but, briefly, until a child is three years old or so his parents notice mainly that he is learning to talk and they are pleased by what they hear. About the time he is three they begin to feel that he *has* learned — and so they are more inclined to notice whether or not he has learned to speak well. It is at this age, therefore, that they may become critical of his speech if they have any tendency to be critical. Moreover, if they are not critical of the child's speech at this time it is not very likely that they ever will be.

It was a related finding, and a very important one, that all forty-six children in the clinical group were said to have spoken without stuttering for several months or even one or two years or more before they were judged to be stutterers. Half or more of the parents said the problem did not arise until about two years after the child had spoken his first words, or a little over one year after he had spoken his first sentences. This naturally suggested a new look at the widely held notion that some children start to stutter as soon as they start to talk. A review of textbooks and technical journals did not turn up any detailed and descriptive accounts of observations of the speech of specific children that would support such an idea. At any rate, our data seemed to indicate that a child is most likely to be classified as a stutterer — if he is ever going to be — when he is two and a half to four years old. This means, of course, that for a year or two he will have talked normally, or at least without anyone thinking he was stuttering, before his parents decide he is beginning to stutter. Any such child does, in fact, demonstrate for a year or so, or even a longer period, that he has whatever it takes to talk without stuttering — or, without being looked upon as a stutterer. Why, then, does he not continue to demonstrate this?

One of the most sobering things we noted in Study I was that the children in the clinical group had been "diagnosed" as stutterers by laymen — nearly always their parents — who, of course, were not trained in speech pathology. What exactly had the children been doing when their parents first got the idea they were beginning to stutter? In all forty-six cases the main kind of speech behavior that the parents had originally taken to be stuttering was described by them as apparently effortless, simple, and generally brief repetitions

45

of the first syllables of words, or of whole words, or phrases. In forty-two of the forty-six cases these were the only things reported by the informants in describing what they called the very first stutterings. The parents thought that the children had not been conscious of these repetitions. Evidently the youngsters were not bothered by what they were doing.

We were frankly puzzled by these reports. The parents did not seem to be talking about the tense, overly hesitant, and emotional speech reactions that we customarily called stuttering. It was not long, however, before we became keenly conscious of the fact that no one had any norms for fluency of childhood speech, or even adult speech for that matter. We simply did not know how fluently, or disfluently, young children speak. In other words, we didn't know whether the parents were talking about kinds of speech reactions that were unusual or ordinary.

This called for action, and we were soon at work on the job of trying to find out how often sounds, words, and phrases are repeated by young children generally in their everyday talking. We did several studies of the speech of the children, from two to five years old, who were attending the University of Iowa Preschools. The first study, done as a Ph.D. thesis by one of my students, Miss Dorothy Davis, sampled the spontaneous speech of sixty-two youngsters in the playrooms and on the school grounds. The average child was found to repeat the first syllables of words, or whole words, or phrases 45 times every 1,000 running words. It did, indeed, seem that what the parents described as their children's very first "stutterings" were primarily quite ordinary kinds and amounts of speech repetition.

We began to realize, therefore, that just because a parent had decided that a child was beginning to stutter we could not be sure that the child was actually beginning to speak in an unusual way. Now, this was most unsettling. In none of the books published up to that time had it ever been suggested that at the moment a child is said to be stuttering for the first time he may, as a matter of fact, be talking quite like other children! And yet from our findings it seemed undeniable that this could very well be the case. Nothing in my professional training had prepared me to take this in stride.

The problem appeared as a rule to have come into existence at the moment the parents first decided the child was stuttering. From that point, the problem took a certain course. In the usual case, what happened was that the child began after a while to talk a little less, and at least at times a bit more hesitantly, with a little more repetition. But the child spoke better sometimes than at other times, and there were periods when the parents thought he was speaking normally. In other words, the problem appeared to "come on gradually." It did "come on," however. It slowly became more serious, not only for the parents but for the child too, with occasional sudden turns for the worse and for the better, or with gradual ups and downs. In the average case between five and six months had passed before the child was brought to our attention, and although many of the youngsters were speaking quite well when we first saw them — indeed, some were speaking normally so far as we could judge — there were some who were talking with definitely more tension and considerably more hesitation and repetition than most children.

◆ ◆ ◆

Although the histories of the children in Study I were impressively similar in basic pattern, the details of each story were more or less distinctive. For example, there was little Johnny Blake from Sioux City. Johnny was not quite three when his father noticed one evening that once in a while he repeated a sound or a word. His father, like so many others, had never done any reading about childhood speech development, or paid any particular attention to the fluency with which children talk. He had been happily conscious of the fact that Johnny had been learning to talk during the past year or two, but it was not something that he had observed closely.

So, when he happened to notice that Johnny now and then repeated a sound or a word, it didn't occur to him to wonder how Johnny compared in this respect with other children of his age. As far as we could make out from the father's account — and in this case we got the story within a week after the events took place, while memories were unusually fresh — he assumed that this was something Johnny had never done before. Meanwhile, if Johnny had not been repeating syllables and words and phrases since he spoke his first word — and if before that he had not repeated something like half of his infant vocalizations — he would have been very different from other children.

Once he got around to noticing Johnny's repetitions, however, Mr. Blake immediately made a mental note to do something about them. The very next morning he just happened to meet the Blakes' family doctor on his way to work, and he said something to the doctor that was understandable and yet most unfortunate. Not realizing apparently that it would make any difference how he worded what he had to say, he did not say simply and quite accurately that Johnny had repeated some syllables and words the evening before. He said instead that Johnny had begun to stutter, and he asked the doctor what should be done for it.

This was indeed a loaded question. Mr. Blake, however, didn't seem to realize that it was loaded. He apparently took for granted that "stuttering" meant the same thing as "repeating syllables and words." It evidently never entered his head that he had, in fact, made a diagnosis. But this was what he had done, of course. He had not made a simple description of the way Johnny had been speaking. He had instead made a very important classification of the speaking Johnny had done.

In telling about this case, I am, for the sake of clarity, getting far ahead of our story. As a matter of fact, it was many years later before I felt that I understood very well what Mr. Blake had done. What I did understand more or less was that when Mr. Blake told the family doctor that Johnny had begun to stutter, the information he gave the doctor was not mainly about Johnny.

"Stuttering," you see, was the name for the judgment that Johnny's father had made of what he had heard Johnny doing. So, what Mr. Blake had given the doctor was some information about himself, about what he himself had thought about Johnny's speech — or some aspect of it. He had not described the way Johnny had spoken.

What is more, the doctor did not seem to understand what Mr. Blake had — and had not — told him. Evidently he had not noticed that Mr. Blake had not described Johnny's speech, but had only indicated how he had classified it. So he did not ask Mr. Blake, "What do you mean by 'stuttering'?" He did not ask for a description of what Johnny had been doing. He simply said that if Johnny was stuttering he should be told to take a deep breath before starting to speak. It is most unlikely that he had any idea what was going to come out of this innocent and well-meant advice.

What did happen was that Johnny's father went home and proceeded, like the conscientious father he was, to do his very best to carry out the advice he had been given. He told Johnny to take a deep breath before trying to speak. Within forty-eight hours the deep breath had become a pronounced gasping — and Johnny was nearly speechless! His mother and father were worried sick.

This was how the problem called stuttering came into being in the very real case of Johnny Blake and Johnny's parents. It was a problem for Johnny's father before it was for Johnny — but almost as soon as his father began to do something about "the problem," Johnny responded in such a way that he had a problem, too. For Johnny the developments were sudden and dramatic. What took place, however, seems to be essentially what happens, more gradually and in other and less dramatic ways, in most cases.

As soon as we arrived on the scene in response to the parents' request for help, we "called off the dogs" and reassured Johnny's parents. We gave them some information about the realities of childhood speech. We left them with a little advice. In due time the parents' feeling about Johnny's speech returned to normal — and so did Johnny's speech.

❦   ❦   ❦

In the case of Billy Wayne, to select a different kind of story, nothing much ever did happen. It was a mighty interesting case though. I had been asked to speak on the subject of stuttering to a club in a nearby town. About a week later a gentleman came to my office, introduced himself as Mr. Wayne, and said his little boy Billy, aged three, was beginning to have some speech trouble. He went on to explain that after he had heard my talk he had gone home and paid more attention to his own boy's speech! He had never paid much attention to it before, he said. What he had observed had bothered him. He had noticed, he said, that Billy was stuttering.

I arranged to visit the Waynes in their own home. I wanted to see Billy and the family together. Billy had a younger sister, and the mother and father and two children lived in a modest, attractive house on a tree-lined street in a pleasant town in Iowa. The house was conspicuously clean and neat, and the yard was well kept. The mother and father were college graduates, and the father was a partner in a successful business. The Waynes were obviously interested in the welfare of their two children.

Indeed, as the story unfolded I began to suspect that they might be somewhat overly concerned about their children. My suspicions were rather well confirmed, I thought, when the mother told me about the methods she was using in toilet training Billy. She explained that she was following a schedule, placing him on the toilet at regular intervals, and keeping him there "as long as necessary." Sometimes, she said, she would give him his lunch or dinner while he was on the toilet, so that he would be there when he needed to be. I gathered that she was also trying hard to teach Billy to be neat and clean and to have good manners. The parents were also watching carefully to see that Billy ate what they thought he should.

In fact, when I asked what Billy had been doing at the time they had first thought he was beginning to stutter, one of the incidents they described had happened at the family dinner table. It seems that Billy had eaten a piece of chocolate cake for dessert and he had asked for a second piece. They had felt it would not be good for him, and so they had refused his request. He asked again. Again, they refused. He persisted. About the fifth or sixth request came out in the form "I I I I I want a piece of cake!"

That, they said, was the first instance of what they called Billy's stuttering. I questioned them very closely, and I satisfied myself that the Waynes were assuming that Billy had never done anything like that before — and that it was not normal for a child to repeat a word in that way under the circumstances they had described.

I asked for more examples of what they had taken to be Billy's stuttering. They were able to remember only one other specific incident. This had occurred when Mr. Wayne was sitting in an easy chair in the living room reading the evening paper, and Billy was standing at the door asking permission to go out. It was raining, and Billy's father said from behind the evening paper that he should not go out because the weather was bad. Again, as in the cake incident, Billy had persisted, and been refused. Finally, Billy had said emphatically, "I I I I want to go out!"

Although they said they thought he had done more "stuttering" than that, those were the only instances they were able to remember. Their concern was real enough, however, and they wanted very much to know what should be done about what they called Billy's stuttering. Even though we had not progressed very far with our studies of speech fluency, I had by this time done enough observing of children's speech to be sure that what the Waynes were telling me about was decidedly commonplace. Any child can be expected to repeat as Billy had done in the kinds of situations the Waynes had described. I did my best to assure them of this, and in the bargain I also tried to persuade them to ease up considerably on the toilet training and somewhat also on the other standards they were applying in bringing up the children. I kept in touch with them over the years and the problem they had about Billy's speech never did become a problem for Billy himself. Apparently the whole family benefited generally from the improved understanding they had gained, and from the relaxing of pressures.

◀   ◀   ◀

These two cases represent the extremes in the development of the problem; most of our other cases, including that of Alice and her mother in Chapter 2, fall between them. Johnny Blake responded to well-meant instructions by beginning quite suddenly to speak with great tension and excessive blocking in addition to — indeed, almost instead of — the simple repetitions characteristic of the normal speech of children of his age. On the other hand, Billy Wayne never did do anything in speaking except what is commonly done by children in situations that are more or less generally experienced by youngsters in American homes. In each instance one or both of the parents first felt that a problem had arisen and they became genuinely concerned about it. Johnny's parents had intervened in a direct way with the child's apparently normal manner of speaking, and the results had been most unfortunate. Even so, since the parents called us quickly we were able to help them reverse the undesirable trends. In the other case the parents had simply worried about what they thought of as something wrong with the child's speech, but they had not done much about it directly. Moreover, they too had sought help promptly, and they made good use of the information and advice they received. The result was that the concern was relieved and a threatening problem was nipped early in the bud.

As the stories of Johnny and Billy suggest, the problems we investigated in our first case studies of the onset of stuttering differed in various ways — and yet, as these stories also suggest, there was a basic pattern of similarity among them. It is not possible, of course, to select two, or twenty, or any other limited number of children who completely represent the variety of youngsters brought to clinics by their mothers and fathers to get help for what they call stuttering. However, the stories of Johnny and Billy illustrate about as well as any two cases might the facts we had gathered up to about 1939 and the most important conclusion we had reached. This conclusion was that what children are doing at the moment someone first thinks they are stuttering is not a kind of "emotional disturbance or instability," or a "breakdown of muscle coordination," or a "disorder of the nervous system." Our data strongly indicated, moreover, that children who are regarded by their parents as stutterers appear to be representative of children generally.

These indications were reinforced in a special way by what we learned when we went back to each "stutterer's" home — two and a half years later in the average case — to see "how things were going." With surprise and pleasure, we found that in about seven out of ten cases the speech was considered by the parents to be normal or "nearly normal." In twenty-five out of the forty-six cases, or 54 per cent, the speech was considered to be normal by all concerned. In five cases everyone agreed that the speech was "nearly normal." In three cases there was disagreement, some holding that the speech was normal while others felt that it was not quite normal. In the other thirteen cases everybody agreed that there was still a speech problem in some degree.

The various judgments obtained may be summarized by saying that in thirty-nine, or 85 per cent, of the forty-six cases improvement or elimination of the problem was reported by the parents; in six it was felt that there had been no important change; and in one the problem was thought to have become worse. During the course of the study, the speech problem had been judged to be severe in six cases, average in twenty-eight, and mild in twelve; at the time of the follow-up, of thirteen cases who were thought still to have a problem, eleven were classified as average, one as mild, and one as severe.

These very encouraging figures are to be viewed with an eye to the sort of help we had given the parents. In general we had tried to get them to think of their youngsters as being capable, physically and in every other way, of normal speech. We had encouraged them to do what they could to make speech more enjoyable and rewarding for the child. We had suggested that they adopt more realistic standards of child behavior so that their youngster could have a fair chance of measuring up to them. We had told them how smoothly — or unsmoothly — they could reasonably expect the child to talk, and explained that he would talk more fluently under some conditions than under others.

In such ways we had tried to get the parents to reduce tensions, both for the child and themselves, and to make it easier for the child to feel success and approval. We had given the parents available information about early childhood speech and the conditions that affect its development favorably and unfavorably. We had also given them information about the onset and development of the problem of stuttering itself. The results of our efforts, as reflected in the follow-up findings, had been decidedly heartening.

◆ ◆ ◆

The data we had gathered could be explained, it seemed to me, only by changing substantially, or by giving up, the only theories of stuttering we had at that time, some twenty-five years ago. But we do not give up our theories, our accustomed ways of thinking, until we clearly see new and better possibilities. Working out a better way of thinking than the ones we have long known, however, is something like developing a new style of painting, or a new form of musical composition. This is by no means simple. And so we did not just sit down one day and make up a brand-new theory of stuttering. The understanding of the problem that we have achieved to date has come slowly, but with each small advance has come greater hope and more encouragement.

CHAPTER 4

Learning to Doubt and Fear

As we carried on our studies beyond 1940 we became more and more confident that we were adding to our facts and our understanding of them. As is true in nearly all kinds of research, however, we found it easier to gather facts than to interpret them. The new information we were getting did not square very well with the old explanations of stuttering that we were used to. We frequently felt a need to look back, as well as ahead, and to take our bearings.

The main facts we had to review and ponder were those that had been gained from several investigations of various kinds from roughly the twenties to the forties, in addition to the case studies we had so far made of the onset of stuttering. These facts made it far easier than it would otherwise have been to change our traditional theories and points of view.

❧   ❧   ❧

The first laboratory investigators of stuttering, both in this country and abroad, approached the problem physiologically. Professor Lee Edward Travis, who began his studies of stuttering in the mid-twenties, was among those who were particularly interested in exploring the possibility that stuttering might be due to some physical flaw in the speaker. In a previously published book (*Stuttering in Children and Adults: Thirty Years of Research at the University of Iowa*, 1955) I have summarized my own impressions of much of the physiological research on the stuttering problem by saying:

"As the years passed, the search for the flaw in the physical make-up of the stutterer changed by degrees from a swift scurry to a slow meander. The simple fact was that the searchers came across other trails in which the scent was warmer. Prolonged and intensive exploration failed, so far as I can judge, to turn up any distinctive physical differences between stutterers and nonstutterers. A few findings along the way caused momentary flurries of excitement, but, as in most other long-term research efforts, experience yielded better and better apparatus, experimental designs, problem formulations, mathematical treatments of data, and basic know-why, and the problems implied in older and cruder findings were consistently dissolved in the refining process. The more skilled and meticulous the investigators became, the more they found stutterers to be, from a neurophysiological point of view, like other people."

The fact that the two groups of children in our first investigation of how stuttering begins were found to be essentially alike with regard to birth conditions, physical development, speech development, general health, and handedness went far in influencing us to think that there probably are no important physical differences between stutterers and normal speakers. In the late thirties and early forties several other studies were completed which gave much additional weight to this view.

At Iowa Professor Charles Strother and Miss Lois Kriegman found no significant differences between young adult stutterers and nonstutterers in the ability to perform rapid or rhythmical movements of the lips, tongue, jaws, and breathing muscles. Their findings were in substantial agreement with those of most earlier studies, but the technical excellence of their work made it specially important in the argument over whether the speech mechanisms of stutterers are normal.

Thirty or more years ago some data were reported which seemed to suggest that there might be certain differences in blood chemistry, especially with respect to calcium and blood sugar, between stutterers and nonstutterers. However, in research in which I worked with Dr. Genevieve Stearns and her staff in the department of pediatrics of the College of Medicine at Iowa (in 1933) no such differences were found between a group of young adult stutterers and comparable nonstutterers. Substantially the same conclusion was reached in a similar study reported (in 1940) by Drs. I. W. Karlin and A. E. Sobel of Brooklyn.

Some of the early studies seemed to suggest possible differences in heart rate and blood pressure between stutterers and nonstutterers, but in 1943 one of my students, Dr. Carl Ritzman, in a carefully designed laboratory study found no notable differences with regard to heart rate, blood pressure, and basal metabolic rate.

In 1944 Dr. Harris Hill, then of the University of Indiana, published in the *Journal of Speech Disorders* two comprehensive reviews of some 150 physiological and biochemical studies of persons classified as stutterers and nonstutterers. After evaluating the data yielded by these many investigations, Dr. Hill concluded that the biochemical changes sometimes found to be associated with stuttering behavior are much the same as those associated with any effortful muscular activity or with emotional reactions following on any frustration and embarrassment. That is, some of the behavior called stuttering is hard work and it gives rise to feelings of uneasiness. It is characterized by the same sort of bodily chemistry as other forms of hard work and emotional concern. There is no special biochemistry of stutterers as persons. Dr. Hill summed up his conclusions on the possibility of a physical cause of stuttering in these words: "An agent in the form of an inner condition . . . is still as distant from discovery as it was 4,000 years ago."

Since about 1925 there had been over a hundred investigations concerned somehow with the question of whether handedness is related to stuttering. As this work progressed the research methods were steadily refined, and what was at first a very confusing picture indeed gradually came into clear focus. As better and better laboratory procedures were used in measuring handedness it became ever more clear that there was probably no solid ground for the so-called handedness or "brain dominance" theory of stuttering. Finally in the early forties three particularly important studies of handedness in relation to stuttering were published. One of these was by Professor Harry Heltman of Syracuse University; the second one was by Dr. E. J. Spadino of Columbia University; and in the third I was associated with Mr. Arthur King. The data from these studies

amounted to an impressive demonstration of the similarity in handedness between stutterers and nonstutterers.

¶   ¶   ¶

Meanwhile, the view that stutterers are in some important way
distinctive in emotionality, or personality, was brought into question
by a number of investigations. One of the earlier of these was a study
I had done between 1929 and 1931 on the influence of stuttering on
personality adjustment. This way of going at it was a departure from
the traditional mode of thinking. The relationship had been stated
previously the other way round, as though personality adjustment or
maladjustment had an influence on stuttering, or on speech, not as
though stuttering influenced personality adjustment. My findings indicated, certainly, that the difficulties and humiliations experienced
by stutterers in speaking to other people affected their social adjustments and their feelings about themselves, but I did not find any
fundamental differences in personality.

The bulk of the work on stuttering in relation to personality adjustment was to be done later, but even by the early 1940's it was
beginning to be fairly clear that so far as anything basic about personality is concerned, stutterers are essentially like nonstutterers.
This is not to say that persons classified as stutterers have no problems of adjustment. It is to say that the problems they do have, while
centering more around speech than is true for most other persons,
are apparently not much more severe or complex than are those of
the general run of people. If there are any differences, they may be
found in a little greater tendency for stutterers to be socially with-
drawing, more or less discouraged about speaking, and somewhat
resentful about their difficulties and disappointments in speaking.
These kinds of group differences cannot always be demonstrated,
however, and there are individual exceptions to them.

It should be noted that such differences in emotional adjustment
between nonstutterers and stutterers as are found in some studies
tend to be, on the average, the right kind and of about the right extent to indicate that stutterers react with normal emotions to their
frustration and humiliation in speaking. They care, but they do not

go all to pieces; and they show a normal capacity for making the best of the fact that they do not always speak as smoothly and easily as other people. They do not appear to differ in adjustment in any deep or basic sense from so-called normal speakers. In 1958 Dr. Leonard Goodstein and Dr. Joseph Sheehan reviewed a considerable mass of research evidence for these conclusions in the *Journal of Speech and Hearing Research* and the *Journal of Speech and Hearing Disorders.*

◀ ◀ ◀

In addition to these more or less traditional studies, in which for the most part comparisons were made between persons classified as stutterers and those classified as normal speakers, a big advance was made during the thirties and forties in working out certain new ways of doing research on the problem of stuttering. These had to do with measuring the changes in amount of stuttering under different conditions. For example, one of the earliest studies I directed concerned the degree to which stutterers speak better or worse in some situations than in others. This study, carried out in 1933 by M. D. Steer, now professor of speech pathology and director of the Speech and Hearing Clinic at Purdue University, was the first of what turned out to be a long series of laboratory investigations in which we sought to answer this very important question: When do stutterers do more and when do they do less of the things that we call their stuttering?

The most important finding that came out of these studies was that when a stutterer reads a passage several times in succession he stutters less and less. We called this the adaptation effect. Professor John R. Knott and I shared the first published report of it in 1937. We found that in reading a passage five times in succession the average stutterer cuts the number of stuttered words by about 50 per cent. Now, it takes the average stutterer only about ten minutes to read a passage of, say, 200 words five times. Whatever is operating to reduce the amount of stuttering by half in ten minutes must certainly be "big medicine." Moreover, the same sort of thing seems to be operating in the daily experience of stutterers, because they tend to talk better to persons and in situations as they become more accustomed to them. The conclusion suggested by these findings is that the more a stutterer talks the better, and the more people he talks to and the more different situations he talks in the better.

One of the questions about stuttering in which I became very much interested was whether it occurred more in saying some sounds and words than others. In the early thirties the opportunity to bring about some research on this was realized when Spencer F. Brown, then a graduate student at Iowa, undertook a study in which a group of stutterers read over 300,000 words. These words were carefully edited so that a suitable tally could be made of stuttering on the different speech sounds and on various kinds of words. Dr. Brown, who is now on the faculty of the Yale School of Medicine and a practicing pediatrician, went far beyond our original investigation to do an extended series of studies. He was able to show that stuttering occurs more on long words than on short ones, more on words that begin with consonants than on words that begin with vowels, and more on the first three words of a sentence than on those in other positions in the sentence. What is perhaps most intriguing of all, he also found that more stuttering occurs on nouns, verbs, adjectives, and adverbs than on words representing other parts of speech. A moment's reflection will suggest that these most frequently stuttered words are the ones that carry most of the meaning of a sentence. Dr. Brown also found that more stuttering occurs in reading a meaningful passage than in reading nonsense material. This last finding was confirmed a few years later (in 1945) by Professor Jon Eisenson and Miss Esther Horowitz of Queens College.

In another study, one of my students, Mrs. Harriet von Krais Porter, determined in 1939 that the more listeners a stutterer has the more he stutters. Her stutterers did more stuttering to two listeners than to one, more to four listeners than to two, and still more to eight. She also observed that stuttering increased when a stutterer read to a listener whom he had rated in advance as "hard to read to" and that it decreased when he read to a listener whom he had rated in advance as "easy to read to."

(These findings seemed especially fascinating because they suggested the possibility — farfetched as it would surely seem to the practical-minded — of a curious new approach to personnel selection in industry or in public agencies. For example, suppose you want to hire a department store manager. According to the data just described, you could proceed by having stutterers read to your applicants one at a time — and then presumably you would hire the one to whom they stutter the most, since he would be shown by such a test to be the most imposing. On the other hand, in employing a nurse or kindergarten teacher presumably you would hire the applicant to whom they stutter the least, since she would seem to be the most understanding. I have no illusions that this procedure is going to replace the methods now in favor, but I feel there might be more than a whimsical basis for my persistent suspicion that someone will find it useful sometime somewhere.)

Mrs. Naomi Berwick, another of my students, once carried out a most unusual set of observations of the speech behavior of stutterers. She asked each of several adult stutterers to give her the name of a person to whom he felt it would be very difficult for him to speak. Then, without the stutterer's knowledge, she obtained a front-view photograph, five by seven inches in size, of each of these listeners. Several days later she asked each stutterer to read aloud to her a 250-word passage five times in succession. As we have previously noted, when a stutterer reads a passage several times in succession he stutters less and less, and on the average the decrease amounts to about 50 per cent in five readings. After the fifth reading in each case, Mrs. Berwick placed in front of the stutterer the photograph of the person to whom he had said it would be hard for him to speak. She asked him to read the passage again — to the photograph. The downward trend was reversed and now the stuttering increased an average of 20 per cent! What's in a picture? Whatever was in Mrs. Berwick's pictures that affected her stutterers must have been "put there" by them, and this is the most important conclusion suggested by her data. In a rather simple but dramatic way this study demonstrated that the stutterer's hesitancy and tension in speaking to a person — even to the person's picture — depends on how he feels about the person.

We have made a great many other studies of the conditions under which stuttering varies. I should like to tell you briefly about three.

61

In 1937 Mr. Leonard Rosen and I attempted to check up on the commonly reported observations that stutterers can sing, or speak slowly, or whisper, and so on without their usual difficulty. Under laboratory conditions, we did find that there was no stuttering during singing and very little while speaking in time to a metronome (saying one word to each beat), or in a "singsong" rhythm, or in a very loud voice, or in a very soft voice, or in a high-pitched voice, or while whispering, or speaking very slowly (a few stuttered less when they spoke more rapidly than usual), or while reading in chorus with a normal speaker. Even two stutterers could read together without stuttering!

Another of my students, Dr. Virginia Barber Simmons, extended these findings in a subsequent and more elaborate investigation. She found that stutterers were able to read aloud without stuttering not only in time to a metronome, but also in time to walking, to a gentle tap on the shoulder, and to a flashing light (saying one word to each beat, step, tap, or flash). In addition, she determined not only that stutterers could read in chorus with others, either normal speakers or stutterers, but that they could do this even while reading different materials, one reading from one book and the other from another book. They did quite well, in fact, even when reading aloud in the presence of loud noise, which an assistant made by banging a large metal wastebasket.

This last observation particularly intrigued me. I refined the procedure and directed a subsequent study, in 1946, in which Mrs. Mary Lou Sternberg Shane had stutterers read while receiving very loud noise through earphones. The noise was so loud that they were completely or almost unable to hear their own voices. Under this condition most of them did not do any stuttering at all and none did very much. In 1956 Dr. Colin Cherry and his associates in England published data which confirmed this observation. We also demonstrated the phenomenon in 1954 in a film, "New Hope for Stutterers," made for a television series, *The Search*, by the Columbia Broadcasting Company, and now available through Young America Films, Inc. It is indeed thought-provoking to see in this film a severe stutterer suddenly start reading very fluently when the noise fed to him through earphones is turned up. It is about as convincing a demonstration as one could imagine of the basic physical ability of stutterers to speak normally — if indeed any further demonstration of this were needed when it has been shown that stutterers can sing, read aloud in chorus with nonstutterers, even with other stutterers (even, indeed, when reading different materials), and speak all right under many other conditions. Stutterers, with few and minor exceptions, talk quite all right, for example, when they are all by themselves.

⁌ ⁌ ⁌

This account would not be complete, of course, without reference to the fact that there are a number of authorities who would not entirely agree with the point of view expressed. There are writers in the field of speech pathology, and in related fields, who contend that what they call stuttering does begin, at least sometimes, with a "breakdown" of the speech function, and that it is caused, at least in some cases, by a physical flaw or an emotional instability. What they appear to mean by "stuttering" is a relatively unusual lack of fluency. I take for granted that everyone who has studied the matter agrees that there are normal kinds and amounts of disfluency, and that children generally, as well as adults, speak with more than ordinary lack of fluency, and with tension, for many different reasons. These reasons range from brain damage, high fever, and extreme fatigue to emotional distress of various sorts, excitement, and simple confusion or "loss for words." We need to be very clear, however, about the fact that not everyone who speaks hesitantly, with repetitions, even with tension, has the particular problem called stuttering. Nor does everyone who has the problem speak with unusual disfluency. The causes of disfluent speech are not, therefore, the same necessarily as the causes of the problem of stuttering.

A book which presents a general picture of the various uses that are made of the word "stuttering," and the correspondingly varied clinical approaches to the things represented by the word, is *A Handbook on Stuttering for Professional Workers*, written by Oliver Bloodstein with the cooperation of ten other authorities on stuttering. The book was prepared under the sponsorship of the American

Speech and Hearing Association at the request of the National Society for Crippled Children and Adults, publishers of the book. A booklet which is distinctive because it was written cooperatively by eight different authorities on stuttering, and represents their agreement with respect to clinical methods for adults, is *Stuttering and Its Treatment*, published by the Speech Foundation of America, Memphis, Tennessee. A book that presents a sampling of current theories is *Stuttering: A Symposium*, edited by Professor Jon Eisenson and published in New York by Harper and Brothers. It contains discussions of the subject by each of six authorities, with a foreword which I contributed at Professor Eisenson's request on the general subject of "why experts disagree."

I don't think experts on the problem called stuttering disagree mainly because they have different kinds of information available to them. They all have access to more or less the same total body of knowledge. I think they disagree chiefly because of differences in training and temperament, in their preferred definitions, their methods of investigation, their "theories about how theories are made," and the basic patterns of language which they use in thinking about the problem.

Meanwhile, as a writer I feel obligated to make as clear to you as I can, without going into distracting detail, just what the data are from which I draw the particular conclusions that, in my judgment, are to be drawn as of this date.

◀ ◀ ◀

While the studies previously described were being carried on in the thirties and early forties some important developments in clinical methods were taking place. In 1928 the psychologist Knight Dunlap, in a book entitled *Habits: Their Making and Unmaking*, had set forth the idea that one way to break a bad habit is to practice doing it deliberately, "on purpose." He tried out this idea at the University of California at Los Angeles in working with a few stutterers, instructing them to perform "on purpose" the things they did when they stuttered. He felt that the results had been promising.

Professor Dunlap's idea was taken up almost immediately by Professor Bryng Bryngelson at the University of Minnesota. On the basis of Dunlap's idea, Professor Bryngelson developed a procedure that he called "voluntary stuttering." He instructed the stutterer to repeat freely and voluntarily the first sound or syllable of a word a number of times before going on to say the word. Sometimes he had the stutterer read aloud for a while, producing every word in this fashion. At other times the "voluntary stuttering" was performed only occasionally in speaking or in oral reading. Some of the "voluntarily stuttered" words were those that the stutterer felt he could say normally and others were those on which he felt he was going to stutter. Professor Bryngelson was encouraged by the results he observed in the first several cases with whom he used this procedure.

He brought the idea with him to Iowa when he came to complete his studies for the Ph.D. degree in 1931. He also brought with him a young man, Charles Van Riper, who stuttered severely, and throughout the year he worked intensively with Van, as he came to be known by all his friends. Dr. Bryngelson insisted that Van "stutter voluntarily" a great deal every day. The results were indeed heartening in the case of Charles Van Riper — who went on himself to achieve the Ph.D. degree in speech pathology and to become one of the leading authorities on stuttering and other speech disorders in the United States.

In 1932 I began to make use of "voluntary stuttering" and by 1934 I was doing the best speaking I had ever known — at least since my early childhood before I came to be regarded as a stutterer. I did not understand very well what I was doing, though, and so I made what seemed to be a serious mistake. I made the mistake because the basic idea of "stuttering on purpose" held tremendous fascination for me and the other stutterers in the Iowa Clinic at that time, and so we tried to figure out all the possible ways we could do our stuttering "on purpose." I decided, with some encouragement from Dr. Van Riper and my other friends in the clinic, to push my luck in this respect as far as I could. The idea was that whenever I felt that I was stuttering I was to stop whatever I seemed to be doing, and then immediately go on to finish the word. What I was trying to do was to come as close as I could to eliminating the stuttering by "voluntarily"

65

stopping the stuttering as soon as I started, and then going on talking immediately.

At first, I was able to do this quite well, but as the weeks went by I found that I was stopping much more than I was going ahead, and I finally reached a point in the spring of 1935 when I was hardly going ahead at all and was almost speechless. I hadn't done anything to change my basic belief that "I was a stutterer" and "couldn't help stuttering," and so my effort to stop doing anything I took to be stuttering became a more or less constant struggle "to keep from stuttering" — a sort of running fight with myself. The struggle became intensely distressing and most baffling, and finally Dr. Travis suggested that I declare a week's moratorium on talking, take a fishing trip with my wife, and give myself time to collect my wits before continuing with my clinical research. I followed his advice — but both my wife and I have since had not the slightest doubt that the last person in the world to go on a fishing trip with is someone who is deliberately observing a week of silence!

For the next several years I carried on a most curious investigation. I think I must have had all the sensations of a cat trying to find its way out of a puzzle box. I was trying to figure out "the best way to do my stuttering." My almost constant companion in this "Project Stuttering Modification" was Dr. John Knott, who also stuttered, and who went on to become a noted brain wave specialist. He is a former president of the International Society of Electroencephalography and director of the Electroencephalographic Laboratory in the department of psychiatry at Iowa. We spent many a long afternoon and evening talking with each other and analyzing in very great detail the things we did when we stuttered. We made copious notes, and we mustered all our ingenuity in an effort to figure out the most effective ways to modify our stuttering behavior. During those years I am sure we "stuttered on purpose" in all the different ways that could be imagined.

We came at last to the conclusion that if you want to interfere with the fluency of your speech there are three basic ways you can do it: you can repeat whole words or parts of words until you "feel like going ahead"; or you can prolong the first sound or posture of a word, again until you "feel like going ahead"; or you can just do nothing, simply pause, while holding the breath — or breathing — as though "waiting for the light to turn green." If you observe closely what it is that adult stutterers do that makes their speech different from that of other persons you will notice that they do one or the other of these three things, or some combination of them. We felt that we greatly increased our understanding of the problem of stuttering by this discovery and by all the intense self-exploration that led up to it.

◀ ◀ ◀

The basic fact revealed by these laboratory and clinical studies was that the behavior called stuttering is extremely modifiable. It is possible for a speaker to change drastically the things he does that he calls his stuttering. He can even do what he regards as stuttering easily and calmly, simply repeating or prolonging sounds, or just pausing. In fact, so far as I know, there is no physical or psychological reason why he should not be able to modify his speech behavior so much that he need not do any of these things, except as they are done by normal speakers. By 1945 or so I had personally worked the new data into my thinking enough to believe that persons who are classified as stutterers are not distinctively different, either physically or psychologically, from persons classified as normal speakers. I was quite sure by that time that what they do when they speak that is different from what is done by normal speakers is made up of the things they have learned to do — strategies, they might be called — in the attempt to "control the stuttering" or "to avoid stuttering." It had come to seem obvious that the reactions called stuttering do not behave like physical symptoms such as boils or fevers. Instead, they are things the stutterer does in response to the sorts of cues — such as specific sounds or words or features of situations — that are essentially like the stimuli for certain other kinds of learned responses.

The idea that stuttering is learned behavior, and not a disorder of muscle function, or a symptom of nervous instability, or of emotional maladjustment, did not come easily, and there are many people who do not yet accept it. They think it is simply ridiculous that anyone would learn to do anything as disagreeable as stuttering. Also, learning implies teaching, and at first thought it seems unbelievable that anyone, especially a parent, would teach a child to stutter! It isn't that simple — or that incredible — of course. Nobody deliberately teaches a child to stutter and no child sets out knowingly to learn to be a stutterer.

What does a child learn that makes him do the things and have the feelings that lead him and others to take for granted that he "is a stutterer"? He learns to doubt and to fear, and to do certain things because he feels doubtful and afraid. He learns to doubt that he can talk smoothly enough to please the people he talks to, mainly his parents. He learns to fear what will happen if he doesn't. What this amounts to is that he learns to be afraid that "he will stutter" and that if he does he, along with "the stuttering," will be disapproved. Naturally, therefore, he learns to do anything and everything he can think of "to keep from stuttering." Instead of just talking he tries to talk "without stuttering" by doing things like pressing his lips together tightly, or holding his breath — but these are the things he does that he, and everyone else, call his stuttering. Stuttering, then, is what the stutterer does trying not to stutter. That is what he learns to do. And he learns to have distressing feelings about it and about himself and other people because of it. He doesn't intend to learn and nobody deliberately tries to teach him any such things, of course. It is just that the way others react to his repetitions and hesitations in speech, and the way he reacts to their reactions, make it likely that he will learn to do and to feel what, in fact, he ends up doing and feeling.

CHAPTER *5*

The Children

IT WAS 1948 before we got round to extending the investigations of the onset of stuttering that we had started in 1934. In the meantime, as was indicated in the last chapter, we had gained much new information and we had learned to think about the problem in new ways. We had, as a consequence, a much better idea than before of the questions still to be asked. We were able to put together a very comprehensive interview of over 800 questions to be answered by mothers and fathers who felt that their children had begun to stutter. We planned to put the same questions to parents who regarded their children's speech as normal, and then make comparisons. We were to be further aided in our work by the fact that since 1934 certain tests, such as the Minnesota Multiphasic Personality Inventory, had been made available, and tape recording had been well developed.

We set to work with our new ideas and new procedures to gather a much larger mass of data than we had accumulated in the thirties on the question of how the problem called stuttering begins. This time we knew more exactly what we wanted to look for, but still we had no idea that we were going to turn up many of the things we were about to discover.

Frederic L. Darley, later to become director of the Speech Clinic, University of Iowa, joined us in time to carry the brunt of the research on the onset of stuttering that we did between 1948 and 1952. He did most of the work in constructing the new elaborate interview, and he collected the data in what we called Study II. In this study Dr. Darley interviewed and tested fifty sets of parents each of

69

whom had decided that a child of theirs had begun stuttering and, with assistance from Miss Sara Conlon and Mr. Robert Higginbotham, fifty sets of parents who regarded their children as normal speakers.

In general, his findings confirmed those of Study I, although they were, of course, much more extensive. They also convinced us that we should pursue the problem still further, and so from 1952 to 1957, under a grant from the Louis W. and Maud Hill Family Foundation, we carried out Study III, the largest of our investigations of the onset of stuttering. In this third study we interviewed each of the fathers and mothers of 150 children regarded, by their parents, as stutterers and of 150 youngsters considered, by their parents, to be normal speakers. In our three studies there were 246 children classified as stutterers, 178 boys and 68 girls, and a like number classified as nonstutterers.

The families in both Studies II and III were matched in social and economic status, and each child in the "clinical" or stuttering group was paired for sex and age with a child in the "control" or nonstuttering group. In both studies we used the same principle we followed in Study I, which was reported in Chapter 3, accepting into the stuttering group any child whose parents regarded him as a stutterer and for whom the parents were seeking clinical help. We made a special effort to include only cases in which the problem was of recent origin. In Study III, in which we collected most of our data and which I shall draw upon most in the pages ahead, the average interval between the onset of the problem and the interview was about eighteen months; in Study II the average interval was a little over four years. The children in Study III were from two to eight years old, the average being five years; they were a little older than those in Study I and somewhat younger than those in Study II. The families were drawn mostly from Iowa, Minnesota, and Illinois, although many of the control group in Study II were from the Washington, D.C., area and New England, and the total of nearly 1,000 parents and 500 children in the three studies represented in varying degrees most regions of the United States.

If you feel that your child has begun to stutter, and if you are concerned about him and are wondering what "might be wrong with him," it is almost certain that your curiosity will enjoy a brisk run through the account, in the pages ahead, of the findings from our intensive investigations of how the problem called stuttering began in nearly 250 cases. In order to keep the account as uncomplicated and readable as possible, it will be limited to Study III, the main investigation, unless reference is made specifically to Study II or Study I. The findings are presented in some detail, because not only are many of the specific facts important to those concerned with the problem of stuttering, but they are also "as interesting as a gossip column" to anyone who wonders, as everybody does, of course, just how other folks behave when they don't have company for dinner.

◆　◆　◆

First of all, if, in spite of what you have read in Chapter 3, you ever wonder whether your child talks the way he does because he might have been injured at birth, you have good reason to set your mind at rest. In Study III the birth histories were practically the same for both groups. The average birth weights were exactly the same, 7.4 pounds, and five children in each group weighed less than 5.5 pounds.

The data concerning duration of labor varied some from study to study in our research program. In Study I the mean duration of labor was a bit longer for the mothers in the control group than it was for those in the stuttering group, in Study II there was essentially no difference between the two groups, and in Study III the mothers of the stuttering group reported a mean duration of labor of a little over eleven hours as compared with the control group mean of nine hours. Both of these mean values are within normal limits. In general, there did not appear to be any real difference between the two groups.

Unusual conditions associated with birth were rare in both groups, but a few more of those that did occur were reported by the control group mothers. The unusual conditions referred to included injuries and falls experienced by the mother during pregnancy, injuries to the baby at birth, presence of cyanosis (blueness of the baby) at birth, difficulty in initiating breathing, umbilical cord around the neck, in-

71

fant unusually quiet, jaundice, convulsions, and slow or weak pulse following birth.

It is significant that there were no group differences in the number of children in whom physical impairments were noted at or shortly after birth, or the number who experienced feeding problems soon after birth, or the amount of crying during the first days of life.

Although the conditions associated with birth were much the same for both groups, there appears, even so, to have been a tendency for the stuttering group mothers — those who thought of their children as stutterers — to experience more concern over the birth of their children. For example, although more illnesses were reported by the control group mothers, a larger number of them than of the clinical group mothers said that they thought their health had been good during pregnancy. Slightly more of the clinical group mothers indicated that they had been upset and had not always been able to eat regularly and retain food during pregnancy. Actually, however, it was the control group mothers who seemed to have had a little more reason for anxiety concerning birth; a greater number of them indicated variations from the expected nine months' duration of pregnancy, and a few more of them reported premature deliveries, induced labor, and unusual conditions associated with childbirth.

The clinical group mothers seemed to feel more conflict about having children, as indicated by the fact that they had had fewer children than the control group mothers (348 to 412) and more only children (25 to 15). Similar findings were obtained in Study II. Another finding that may have indicated somewhat greater uneasiness on the part of the stuttering group mothers was the fact that they did not breast-feed their babies as long as did the mothers in the control group.

The differences between the two groups were not black and white, however. For example, similar responses were made by both groups of parents to such items as these: "Was the child planned?" "Was the child wanted by both of you?" "Did you or the other parent hold the child during bottle feeding?" "Do you expect to have any more children?"

The findings can be fairly summarized by saying that the two groups of mothers appeared to differ somewhat on reports of conditions of birth, but the facts concerning the children themselves seemed to be quite similar for both groups.

◀ ◀ ◀

Has it occurred to you that maybe your child speaks as he does because he is not well coordinated, or that possibly his handedness has had something to do with it?

With respect to bodily coordination, the similarities between the two groups of children far outweighed the very few minor differences that were suggested. In fact, the differences were of interest mainly because they were so slight and apparently insignificant. All they amounted to was that the control group children had better coordination in catching, as rated by their mothers though not by their fathers, and in running and jumping, as rated by their fathers though not by their mothers — and more stuttering group youngsters, according to the mothers but not according to the fathers, very much preferred the right hand when they first used a pencil or crayon.

There were apparently no significant differences in coordination between the two groups of children in throwing, drawing and coloring, writing, cutting, and manipulating blocks and tinker toys and beads, and in other tasks requiring manual dexterity. There were also no significant differences in the youngsters' original hand preference in using a spoon and in their present hand preference in using a pencil, crayon, or spoon. Both groups made the same median score on a handedness questionnaire filled out for each child by his parents. Both groups were predominantly right-handed. Approximately one third of the children in both groups had learned to write, and very few in either group had shown "a tendency to write backwards." All the data concerning handedness showed the two groups of children to be very similar.

◀ ◀ ◀

Do you have a question about your child's rate of development, or his health and medical history?

The average age at which the children accomplished the following kinds of development, as reported by their mothers, revealed no sig-

73

nificant differences between the two groups: first tooth, full set of twenty baby teeth, creeping or crawling, sitting up unsupported, taking first steps alone, voluntary control of bowels, voluntary control of bladder (day), voluntary control of bladder (night), and using spoon in feeding.

The information obtained concerning the health and physical condition of the children also indicated that the two groups were very similar. They were almost exactly alike in average weight and height.

We made a particularly comprehensive study of the children's illnesses. The average numbers of illnesses were 2.9 and 2.8 for the clinical and control groups, respectively. The clinical group mothers seemed to have paid more attention to the illnesses of their children, however, and they remembered them more vividly, particularly the ones the youngsters had had during their very early years. More of the mothers in the control group had a rather casual attitude toward the illnesses of their children and were unable to remember exactly when they had had particular diseases. More of them were unable to remember which disease a child had had at a particular time.

There were no real differences, meanwhile, between the two groups of children in frequency of colds, their appetites, the amount of energy possessed by the children as rated by their parents, and the numbers for whom constipation was reported. About the same number of children in each group had undergone surgical operations.

The clinical group parents seemed to be somewhat more fussy over their children's illnesses, real or fancied or exaggerated, and to worry more about their health. For example, more of them said that when their children were ill they "fussed over" them and "spoiled and indulged them excessively." Again, although the two groups of children seemed equally healthy, and were rated similarly by their parents with regard to the amount of energy which they seemed to have, nevertheless more of the stuttering group mothers felt that their children tired more easily than the average child. Too, although fewer of the clinical group parents said their children slept very well, actually both groups of children slept the same number of hours per night, on the average, according to the parents.

The data suggest that children classified as stutterers are not in any distinctive way different from other children, so far as their physical development and health are concerned. If you regard your child as a stutterer you have good grounds, then, for looking upon him as physically normal unless medical examination does show something to be at fault. If your doctor demonstrates some physical flaw in your child, there is still a question, of course, whether it has anything to do with the way he talks. Certainly, the findings of our research do not provide you with any basis for assuming that there is probably something physically wrong with your child.

◄ ◄ ◄

If you have been wondering whether your child's speech development is normal — aside from anything you think of as stuttering — you will be interested to learn that the children in both our groups were well within normal limits in speech development. Both groups spoke their first words at a mean age of about eleven months, and their first sentences at roughly twenty-one months on the average. Even so, more of the stuttering group mothers rated their children as "much slower than average" in learning to speak, indicating a tendency to judge their children less favorably than the facts seemed to warrant. There were no significant group differences in the parents' ratings of the amount of talking the children did between the ages of one and five years, the children's vocabularies, their grammar, the current amount of talking done by the children, and the amount of talking the children were allowed to do at the dinner table and when guests were present. Although there were a few more in the clinical group who did not always form all their sounds plainly, few children in either group were reported to have serious speech problems other than stuttering.

◄ ◄ ◄

Are you inclined to think there might be some connection between what you call your child's speech problem and his general level of social development or maturity of behavior?

We have already noted that the parents who regarded their children as stutterers also tended to make certain other evaluations of them which were less favorable than the objective data justified. You will remember that the ratings they made of how well their children slept, how easily they became tired, and the rate at which they developed speech were not well supported by related information concerning the number of hours slept each night, the general health and energy level of the children, and the ages at which they had said their first words and sentences.

The indicated lack of agreement between the parents' ratings of the children and the more objective facts about them should be kept in mind in considering what we were able to find out about the social development of the children. Most of our information was obtained by asking the parents how often each of several kinds of behavior occurred, and they responded by using a rating scale which provided for the following answers: much more than average, somewhat more than average, about average, somewhat less than average, much less than average, and uncertain. This rating system was used in responding to such items as "How much does your child daydream?" and "How much does your child play alone?" Another set of ratings involved a choice from among these answers: very often, quite often, occasionally, never, uncertain. The parents used this system of rating in responding to a series of such questions as "How often has timidity occurred during the past month?" and "How often does your child play with companions?"

There were thirty-five items concerning social development on which the control group children were rated more favorably by either their mothers or their fathers, or by both, than were the clinical group children. On seventeen of these thirty-five the mothers and fathers agreed. These seventeen items had to do with such things as daydreaming, playing alone, nervousness, timidity, showing off, rudeness, fear of strangers or other children or the dark, bids for attention, and being laughed at by other children.

Such group differences in parents' ratings of their own youngsters must be interpreted carefully. In fact, it is necessary to use a gray language, so to speak, in discussing practically all the differences between the two groups of children, as well as those between the two groups of parents. Most of the differences are by no means sharply defined. The differences in social development appear to be particularly subtle and generally slight, with much overlapping between the groups. For example, it is interesting to note that more of the stuttering than of the control group fathers — the mothers did not differ — gave their children the most favorable rating possible in response to the question "How does the child adjust to new situations and friends?" This and other related findings suggest that such differences as there may be between the two groups with regard to social development and social adjustment are not extreme.

In this connection it is to be remembered that the responses we are talking about here were made in the form of ratings, and these ratings were made by the parents eighteen months, on the average, after the clinical group parents had first thought their children were stuttering. The ratings may have been affected, therefore, by the parents' concern over their children's speech during this average period of a year and a half. Moreover, the children also may have been affected during this period by the concern and dissatisfaction shown by their parents.

It is also to be considered that the two groups of parents did not differ significantly in rating their children with respect to the following items: the age of their children's friends, the tendency to be mischievous, the ability to concentrate, aggressiveness, carelessness, being picked on at school, popularity, fighting, laughing, respecting the rights of others, bedwetting, hitting other children, crying at home, hurting pets, nail biting, temper tantrums, whining, teasing, bullying, disobedience, explaining away faults, athletic ability, reading, ease of crying, happiness, rivalry, the amount of teasing the children received, the things the children were teased about, stealing, masturbation, playing with sex organs, the child's evaluation of his own abilities, the child's perfectionism about his own speech, strong fears other than those already listed, and the number of organizations to which the child belonged.

It helps to round out the picture to note also that so few parents reported the following that they are not to be considered important in either group: sleepwalking, crying at school, face twitching, fainting, and running away from home.

The majority of the ratings made by the parents in response to all

77

the social development and behavior items were moderate rather than extreme. On most of these items most of the parents rated their children as either about average or somewhat above or somewhat below average. Relatively few parents rated their children as much more or much less than average on these items. In response to the questions concerning the frequency of occurrence of specific kinds of behavior such as nervousness and timidity, the great majority of the answers were "occasionally" or "never," with comparatively few being "very often" or "quite often."

◄　◄　◄

Is your youngster an only child? Or the oldest? Or youngest?

In the control group of 150 children in Study III there were 15 who were only children; 41 were oldest, 53 youngest, and 41 middle children (second, third, fourth, fifth, or sixth in order of birth) in their respective families. For the stuttering group the corresponding figures were 25 only children, and 56 oldest, 45 youngest, and 24 middle children (second, third, or fourth in order of birth). It is to be considered that the oldest child in any family occupies the position of an only child until the arrival of a brother or sister. Therefore, if we combine the only children and the oldest children in each group, it turns out that in the control group 56 (37 per cent) and in the stuttering group 81 (54 per cent) were, or for a time had been, only children. The difference between these two percentages is statistically significant; that is, it is a genuine, not a chance, difference.

When the children from Study II and Study III are thrown together, there are 36 only children out of 200 in the stuttering group and 20 out of 200 in the control groups, and the difference between these figures is also statistically significant.

What is the meaning of the fact that a higher proportion of the children classified as stutterers are only children? A likely answer would seem to be that parents who have only one child are inclined to be particularly concerned over him, to notice a bit more intently how he is getting along, and to pay more attention to any possible shortcomings or illnesses or problems that he may seem to have. This would probably increase the parents' tendency to focus their attention upon the child's speech and to be especially concerned about it.

◀ ◀ ◀

In the literature dealing with the subject of stuttering one finds here and there the statement that stuttering is more likely to be found among twins than other children. It is also said that it is more often true of identical than of non-identical twins that both members of a pair stutter. Research has not always confirmed this, however. Whether or not you are the mother or father of twins, you are probably curious to know what has been scientifically determined.

One of my students, Miss Odny Graf, found in a study of 552 pairs of twins that there was no notable difference between identical and non-identical twin pairs in incidence of stuttering. In one out of seven pairs who were presumably identical both twins stuttered, while in two out of nine non-identical pairs both twins stuttered. Miss Graf found 21 persons, or a little under 2 per cent of her total sample of 1,104 twins, who were said to be stutterers. The percentage of persons in the general population who are classified as stutterers has been reported by different investigators to lie between a little over half of 1 per cent and 2.5 per cent. Probably the most acceptable estimate would place the number a bit under 1 per cent.

The fact that Miss Graf found a slightly larger proportion of twins classified as stutterers makes a kind of sense. Twins are somewhat like only children, in that they may very well be given more attention by their parents than other children. Moreover, it would seem reasonable to suppose that if the parents were to decide that one of the twins is a stutterer they might be rather more than likely to wonder at least whether the other one might be stuttering, too. If this is so, the result would probably be that a slightly larger proportion of twins than of other children are classified as stutterers by their parents.

In Study III there was only one child in the clinical group who was a twin, and there were no twins in the control group. In Study II one child in the control group and two in the clinical group were twins. Thus, of the 200 clinical group children in both Study II and Study III, three, or 1.5 per cent, were definitely members of twin pairs. From available figures, drawn from a considerable number of studies involving a variety of groups or samplings, it would appear that about 1.1 to 1.4 per cent of the general population are twins.

Interestingly enough, in Study III five parents, two fathers and three mothers, in the control group and three parents, two fathers and one mother, in the stuttering group were twins. Moreover, the parents in Study III were asked whether there were any twins among their relatives, and forty-nine relatives of control group parents and forty-one relatives of parents in the stuttering group were reported to be twins.

◀ ◀ ◀

If you feel that your child is stuttering, and you are like most other people, you probably wonder occasionally whether the problem could be due in some way to heredity.

The parents in both groups were asked: "Are there other stutterers in your family?" Nine mothers and eight fathers in the control group and thirty-five mothers and thirty-five fathers in the clinical group gave a yes answer to this question. Of the control group children, three had stuttering parents, all fathers, and, according to the father but not the mother, one had a sibling — a brother or sister — who stuttered. Of the children in the clinical group, nineteen had fathers and five had mothers who stuttered, while seven, according to the fathers, and nine, according to the mothers, had stuttering siblings.

These data are in general agreement with the findings of many other studies that have been reported. They can be explained in at least two ways.

According to the one the problem of stuttering "runs in families," to the extent that it does, because it is biologically inherited. What we inherit, of course, are features of bodily structure, such as color of eyes, texture of hair, contour of face, and general bodily shape. We can apparently inherit physical conditions which tend to lead to deafness, or to deficiencies in vision, or to disturbed functioning of the heart or of other bodily organs. Now, although there has been considerable scientific study of the physiological and anatomical factors that might possibly be related to stuttering, we have not been able to establish that it is due to a flaw in any part of the body, inherited or not. It is exceedingly difficult, therefore, to determine what a child might inherit that would cause anyone to classify him as a stutterer.

The problem is peculiarly complicated by the fact that, as we shall see later, the children who were classified as stutterers and those who were not so classified in our studies were apparently not speaking very differently at the time someone in each case first decided stuttering had begun. But, of course, even if all the clinical group children had been speaking with many more repetitions and hesitations than all of those in the control group, it is not clear that one or more parts of the body would need to have certain characteristics, and if so what these would have to be, in order to bring this about.

It is even more difficult to think that the problem called stuttering might be due to heredity when we consider our finding that the clinical group parents judged the speech of their children to be satisfactory or normal for a considerable period, even a number of years in some cases, before deciding they were stuttering. While there are, of course, hereditary characteristics that do not show up until some time after birth, in this instance due consideration must be given to the manner in which the problem called stuttering has been found to originate, and to the fact that even very brief counseling of the parents resulted in elimination of the problem, or improvement, in a large majority of the cases in our studies. It is to be wondered what a child might inherit that would be wiped out by such a small amount — or, indeed, even by a great amount — of counseling of the child's parents.

There is, as has been suggested, another kind of explanation of the tendency for the problem of stuttering to "run in families" to the extent that it does. According to this, what is passed along within families from one generation to the next are certain attitudes or beliefs that seem to be essential to the development of the problem. That is, in addition to biological or genetic factors, there are others that are social — custom, tradition, training. For example, the Mormon religion, or the Methodist or Buddhist, or any other tends to run in families. We understand, of course, that this is a matter of family tradition, something passed along by parental teaching from generation to generation. Thus we have family traditions with respect to food preferences and dislikes, political leanings, ethical and moral tendencies, and attitudes, beliefs, and evaluations generally.

The reason why stuttering runs in families to the extent that it does seems to be one of tradition rather than genes. Parents who stutter, or have stuttered, or who have grown up with stutterers in their families may be expected, in some cases at least, to react somewhat differently to the normally disfluent early speech of their children from parents to whom stuttering is unfamiliar.

We started a fascinating family study in this connection some twenty years ago and it is still being continued. A student of mine, Mrs. Marcella Gray Cass, was employed in 1939 as a speech correctionist in one of the schools in Iowa. She was asked to hold evening classes for adults who stuttered, and the first class was attended by seven persons, six of whom belonged to the same general family group. We shall call them the Simpsons, although that was not their real name.

It was possible in 1939 to trace the Simpson family back five generations. At that point the story began with a stuttering mother and a nonstuttering father. They had two daughters, one of whom stuttered. The stuttering daughter married a normal speaker and the normally speaking daughter married a stutterer. There were several stutterers among the children of these two couples, and in this generation the family divided. Some of them moved to Kansas and the rest stayed in Iowa. After that the two branches of the family lost touch with each other. In the fourth and fifth generations stuttering flourished in Iowa, but in Kansas it all but disappeared. There was only one stutterer to be found in Kansas in the fourth generation and none in the fifth, but in Iowa three out of nine children of the fourth generation and eight out of twenty-four in the fifth generation — one third of all the children — were regarded as stutterers or as former stutterers. One in the fourth and two in the fifth generation were said to be former stutterers — that is, they were not thought of as stutterers at the time of our study but they had been so considered previously.

There were three especially interesting facts about the Iowa "stuttering Simpsons." One was that most of them were said to have stuttered from the time they first began to talk. It was as though their parents had hovered over the cradle waiting to see if they too were going to stutter. It is well known by now, as we have seen in previous chapters, that any child who is just beginning to say words does a great deal of repeating and anyone who is looking for stuttering, and who thinks of stuttering as consisting of the repetitions of sounds and words, might very well conclude that almost any child is beginning to stutter.

The second of these three interesting facts was that in this family there were not more boys than girls, but rather an equal number of each, classified as stutterers. It was apparently more important for a child to be a Simpson than it was for him to be a boy or a girl, so far as the parents' evaluation of his speech was concerned.

The third distinctive fact about this family was that it was more or less dominated in certain respects by one of its members, who was the leader, or chief, of the comprehensive family group. He was the one whom all the others usually consulted before completing a business deal, getting married, or making any other important decisions. He had pronounced views about stuttering. He was convinced that it was hereditary in the Simpson family. And all the other members of the Iowa branch of the family reflected his views and attitudes concerning stuttering. This man was scarcely known to the Kansas branch of the Simpson family, and so they had not been influenced by his thinking about the problem.

All this was interesting enough, but recently I have had an opportunity to bring our information about the Simpson family up to date. I have not quite completed the current investigation and so I have not yet published a report of it, but I can summarize the main findings in a few words. The Iowa Simpsons were interviewed in their homes by Mrs. Cass about twenty years ago. In addition, some of the members of the family visited the Speech Clinic at the University of Iowa at about that time. As a result of these interviews and clinical conferences they received a considerable amount of information concerning the stuttering problem, and evidently this information influenced their thinking. You will recall that one third of the twenty-four children of the family in the fourth and fifth generations were stutterers or former stutterers. In the sixth generation of Iowa Simpsons, however, not one out of forty-four children has been classified as a stutterer.

I asked one of the members of the fifth generation who is a stutterer, and who is now married and the mother of two normally speaking children, how she would explain the fact that the problem of stuttering is not occurring any more in the Simpson family. She answered quickly and matter-of-factly, "We know now how it started, and we aren't saying anything to the younger generation like they told us when we were little." From her elaborations of this statement and from additional information I have obtained from other informants, I would say that there has been a clear change in the family thinking about stuttering and a corresponding change in parental policies and practices concerning the children's speech. In fact, today's parents in the Simpson family, knowing what the family went through in past generations, appear to be positively determined to make no issue of childhood lapses in fluency, and to lean over backwards in seeing to it that the youngsters who are just learning to speak are not criticized for disfluency.

It takes more than one such study, certainly, to finish off a problem as complex as this one, but the data obtained from this one family are clearly suggestive of a tentative conclusion — that the marked changes in incidence of stuttering from generation to generation, and from Iowa to Kansas, within this family are to be more readily explained as the result of modifications in family attitudes and knowledge, and corresponding child-rearing practices, than as the result of changes in the family genes.

The folk thinking about the problem called stuttering has been, and still is, that stuttering is a disorder of speech, and that the causes of it are to be looked for accordingly within the body, or the personality, of the speaker. In some specific way, therefore, according to this mode of thinking, speakers classified as stutterers should be different from other speakers — different in a way that would account for the fact that they stutter, or that they have come to be regarded as stutterers.

We found, however, that the children in our research program whose parents had decided they were stuttering were much more similar to than different from the children whose parents regarded them as normal speakers.

We also compared the two groups of parents. What we found when we did that is the subject of the next chapter.

CHAPTER *6*

The Parents

THE parents in our studies have been of two kinds, those who had decided that their children were stuttering, and those who thought their youngsters were talking all right. We compared them in many different ways, and within each group we compared the mothers with the fathers in several respects. The findings should give you some important clues to the sort of parent you are — or might have been, or might still become. They will certainly give you a look-in at a great many of the details of American family life, and surely you will end up agreeing that it is fully as interesting as the family life of the Eskimos or the Hottentots or the Australian aborigines.

◀ ◀ ◀

The control group parents, especially the fathers, were slightly older than were those in the stuttering group. Between seven and eight out of every ten of the families in both groups were in the middle and upper socioeconomic classes, although far more were in the middle than the upper class. The proportion of our families who were in these two classes, as contrasted with the lower classes, was considerably larger than would be true of families in the general population. This suggests that stuttering is more likely to be found in the big home on the hill than in the little, run-down house on the wrong side of the tracks — that perhaps it is part of the price we pay for the kind of civilization we have bought.

Important as social class itself probably is, in relation to stuttering, it is probably not as significant as the degree to which the family is "upward mobile" — striving, that is, to better itself by climbing

86

to higher ground socially. This can be stated only as a hunch; more research is needed before a firm conclusion can be drawn. The hunch is consistent, however, with the general pattern of all we have learned so far. The more parents expect of their children, the better impression they want them to make, and the more favorably they want them to represent the family in school, in the neighborhood, and before the public generally, the more likely they are to pay attention to anything that seems to be a shortcoming and to make an issue of it. If in such circumstances the parents focus their attention on the child's speech there is some chance that they will create a problem concerning it.

There was very little difference in social and economic status between our two groups of parents, of course, because we matched them to begin with on the basis of such status. It is particularly interesting, therefore, that in answer to the question, "How well-to-do do you consider yourself to be now?" the control group mothers gave themselves higher ratings than the stuttering group mothers gave themselves. In other words, the clinical group made ratings of their economic circumstances that were less favorable than the facts warranted. Moreover, they did not rate as highly as did the control group parents the degree to which the father's employment made use of his abilities. On a very large number of other related items, however, the two groups did not differ significantly.

◀ ◀ ◀

The control group mothers and fathers — those who were satisfied with their children's speech — seemed to have somewhat more varied social interests than the mothers and fathers who thought their children were stuttering. For one thing, they placed a somewhat higher value on friendships. There were other differences, too. For example, the control group mothers belonged to more organizations and participated more frequently in musical activities. The parents in the control group also held more offices in the organizations to which they belonged. At the same time, however, the clinical group parents gave themselves the higher ratings in response to the question "How easily do you adjust to new situations and new friends?"

They also gave each other higher ratings than did the parents in the control group in answering the question "How easily does your wife (husband) adjust to new situations and new friends?"

Although there were such differences between the two groups of parents, they were also very much alike in other related respects. Some of the items on which they did not differ were these: frequency of attendance at movies, of dancing, of playing cards, of going on vacations, of going to parties, and expressed degree of concern over the impressions made on other people.

So far as these data reveal "social adjustment," the two groups of parents were undoubtedly more alike than different — and although they were a little different, yet they were both, as groups, quite normal. This was also shown by their scores on the Minnesota Multiphasic Personality Inventory, a widely used personality test. This test revealed no notable differences between the groups, and both groups scored generally within the normal range. The difference between the two samples of parents in social adjustment seems to be mainly a matter of a little less self-acceptance, or less satisfaction with their state of adjustment, on the part of the mothers and fathers in the clinical group.

◀ ◀ ◀

It has already been suggested that the many details presented in this part of the book may be "as interesting as a gossip column." As a matter of fact, the universal interest that has made the gossip column a standard part of every newspaper was not wholly neglected in this investigation. We asked a very large number of questions about the marriage relationship in each case. The responses of our two groups of parents to these questions probably reflect quite well the matrimonial state of affairs in this country — or at least those parts of it represented by the parents we interviewed. Agreement and disagreement between husbands and wives in answering the questions indicated their general state of marital adjustment or discord.

Here, as in most other parts of the study, the two groups seemed to be considerably more alike than different. There were, however, a number of interesting differences, and they seemed to indicate that the husbands and wives in the control group were getting along a little better than were those in the stuttering group. The clinical group of mothers and fathers seemed to be a bit more dissatisfied with each other's behavior, as well as the behavior of their children.

Particularly interesting were the answers to the question "How well satisfied are you with your present marital relationship?" The two groups of fathers gave about the same answers to this question, about two thirds of both groups saying they were completely satisfied and only a few in each group indicating a degree of dissatisfaction. The two groups of mothers differed somewhat. It was not that very many in either group were definitely dissatisfied. In fact, only two out of 150 of the stuttering group mothers said they were highly dissatisfied, and none of the 150 control group mothers said they were; only four in each group said they were even moderately dissatisfied. The difference between the two groups lay in the fact that more of the control group mothers indicated complete satisfaction with their present marriage relationship (118 to 96), whereas more of the stuttering group mothers indicated that they were only fairly well satisfied (47 to 28).

How would you answer these two questions: "Do you consider the other parent to be too demanding of the child?" "Do you consider the other parent to have spoiled the child?" More stuttering than control group mothers answered yes to both of these questions. At the same time, the two groups of fathers answered them in about the same way. Approximately one fourth of the stuttering group mothers gave a yes answer to both of the questions. More of the stuttering than of the control group fathers answered yes when asked: "Do you consider the other parent to be too easygoing concerning the child?" Roughly a fourth of the stuttering group fathers answered yes to that question.

These data suggest a certain amount of disagreement over child-rearing policies and practices. No doubt this bone of contention between mothers and fathers is as old as the hills. It may be of some importance that the problem was felt a bit more keenly by the parents in our stuttering group than by those in the control group. This suggests that in homes in which there is a general atmosphere of dissatisfaction and a tendency to disapprove, a child's speech may be more likely to meet with parental disapproval than in a home where there is a little more contentment and acceptance of things as they are.

Here is a particularly pointed question to try out on yourself: "As a general rule how tense are you?" Although the two groups of fathers did not differ significantly, the ratings of the stuttering group mothers suggested more tension than did those of the mothers in the control group. Nearly three out of five of the stuttering group mothers said they were very or quite tense as a rule. About two out of five of the control group mothers said this of themselves. These figures seem to be rather high for both groups, and they suggest that the role of the young mother in our society is emotionally pretty demanding. The corresponding figures for the fathers, incidentally, were lower, but they were high enough to suggest that even the lot of the young father in our culture is, for substantial numbers at least, apparently not a bed of roses. However, due weight is to be given to the fact that two thirds or more of the fathers in both groups said they were "not very" or "not at all" tense as a general rule. When asked, "How tense is your wife (husband)?" the two groups of mothers did not differ in rating their husbands, but the stuttering group fathers rated their wives as more tense than the control group fathers rated their wives.

Here is another pointed question: "How irritable are you?" Very few in either group answered "not at all." Roughly two thirds in both groups said they were "not very" irritable. The rest said they were "very" or "quite" irritable, with those in the clinical group admitting to more irritability by a modest margin.

"How do you think your married life compares in happiness with that of your married friends?" The fathers in the two groups answered this question in about the same way, but more of the control group mothers — about three out of five as against two out of five in the clinical group — considered themselves more happily married than their friends. The fathers in the stuttering group reported more quarreling, but the two groups of mothers gave about the same answers to the question "How much do you quarrel as compared with your married friends?" More of the stuttering than control group fathers (the mothers didn't differ) answered yes to the question "Do you believe that the other parent worries too much?"

These differences between the two groups of parents are to be weighed against the very large number of items on which they did not differ to a statistically significant degree. These items included the following: the extent to which the husbands and wives enjoyed being with each other; the differences between husbands and wives over religion, use of money, amount of social life desired, kind of entertainment and types of friends preferred; attitudes of the wife toward the husband's employment, feelings about in-laws, notions about how to spend vacations, preferences with respect to recreation, political views, and preferred radio and television programs.

It may be said — speaking again in a gray language — that the marriage relationship was marked by a bit more tension and dissatisfaction in the stuttering group than in the control group of parents. What this probably means is that parents who are somewhat tense and discontented are a bit more likely to find fault with the fluency of their children's speech. Finding fault may also make them discontented. It is very hard to state this, however, without overstating it, for many other factors are related to this one.

◄ ◄ ◄

The social atmosphere of the home is an important factor affecting family life. It might be described in many ways, of course. We tried to get at it by asking a series of questions that yielded the following information.

First of all, it is to be said — again — that the two groups of parents gave essentially the same kinds of answers to most of the questions asked in this part of the investigation. They did not differ significantly, for example, in their expressed intention to have more children, the number of wives who worked outside the home, the number of families in which both parents worked during the infancy or early years of the child's life, the frequency with which both parents were home evenings, the number of persons (other than members of the immediate family) who had lived in the home at any one time, and the frequency with which the child met visitors in the home. The two groups of families had gone on about the same number of

91

automobile trips, and they were much alike in their movie-going habits.

Certain questions had to do with how the parents and the child got on together, or with how well the parents agreed or disagreed about various things. For example, the two groups of parents did not differ in the degree to which they believed that a child "should be seen and not heard." They did not differ in preferring boys or girls as children. As many in the one group as in the other indicated that they most enjoyed the particular child included in our investigation (in families having more than one child). The amount of "wholehearted laughing" done by the parents seemed to be about the same in both groups. Also, the two groups were about alike with respect to the amount of time that the mothers and fathers had been separated from their children; half or more of the mothers and fathers in both groups had not been away from their children for more than one month.

What differences there were between the two groups of parents were far from clean-cut. The control group parents rated their neighbors as more friendly than did the parents in the stuttering group — but at the same time the stuttering group mothers gave the higher ratings in indicating how favorably the neighbors treated their children. The control group families more frequently went on picnics, according to the mothers but not the fathers. According to both the fathers and mothers, more of the clinical group families never played parlor and card games together.

Incidentally, how often do you and your youngsters go on picnics together? Only a few of the families in our research samples never did. It may come as a surprise to you, as it did to me, that from seven to eight out of every ten of our families said they went on picnics from once a month to several times a week.

How often does your family play parlor or card games? In our two groups, taking only the answers of the mothers, nearly three out of five in the stuttering group and exactly two out of five in the control group said their families never did. One third of the stuttering group and about half of the control group said they played such games from once a month to as often as every day.

In general, our two groups of homes were considerably alike in their social atmospheres. The relationships between the parents, and between the parents and the children, however, seemed just a little less close in the families of the clinical group than in those of the control group. Again, this may have contributed, at least slightly, to the parents' readiness to be somewhat less accepting of the children's speech. It may also have affected the children so that sometimes at least they may have been a little more hesitant in speaking to their parents.

◄ ◄ ◄

If you are like most other people, you are probably inclined more or less to the view that when things don't seem to be going well for children the general health picture of the family bears looking into. In our investigation, however, the two groups of families appeared to be equally healthy.

Because of certain theories concerning stuttering that have been put forth from time to time, it is of interest that only five parents in the control group and six in the stuttering group reported persons with epilepsy in their families. None of the children in either group had epilepsy. Someone was said to have diabetes in about 15 per cent of the families in the clinical group and 10 per cent of those in the control group. Allergies are apparently more common; about one third of the parents in the stuttering group and somewhat more in the control group reported that one or more members of their families had allergies. None of these group differences was statistically significant — that is, larger than differences that might occur by chance in samples the size of ours.

The two groups of families were practically alike in the ratings of present health of the parents, the number of times that members of the family had been ill, the total time covered by illnesses in the family, and the degree to which the parents worried about getting sick. Nor did the two groups differ with regard to either the parents' or the children's appetites, how well the parents slept, their food dislikes, and the frequency with which the parents used alcohol.

In general, as has been said, our two samplings of families were much the same so far as health was concerned, and they were probably fairly representative of the general population from which they were drawn.

✦ ✦ ✦

We have already discussed the so-called handedness theory of stuttering. In view of the popularity this theory once enjoyed, it is of interest that the two groups of mothers and fathers made almost identical scores on our handedness questionnaires. The two groups of families were alike in handedness even when all blood relatives were included (the child's parents, brothers and sisters, uncles, aunts, and grandparents in each case). Children classified as stutterers, or their families, are not different from other people so far as handedness is concerned, according to our findings.

✦ ✦ ✦

On the whole, both of our groups of parents seemed to share the standards and attitudes concerning child development that are generally characteristic of our culture. The few differences we noted between the two groups, however, are of considerable interest.

All the mothers and the fathers were asked to indicate how soon after birth they thought a child should be toilet-trained, say single words, speak sentences, speak intelligibly, and speak fluently. The mothers in the stuttering group indicated that their standards for the achievement of these abilities were higher than those of the mothers of the control group.

The stuttering group mothers would have a child saying single words four months earlier on the average than the mothers in the control group, and they would have children speaking sentences two months earlier. Both of these differences were statistically significant —larger than chance differences. The stuttering group mothers thought a child should "speak fluently" by the time he is a little over forty-eight months old, as compared with a mean age of a little over fifty-two months set by the control group mothers.

The stuttering group mothers would establish nighttime bladder control almost six months sooner on the average than would the more lenient mothers in the control group, and they believed that daytime bladder control, as well as bowel control, should be achieved nearly three months sooner than the control group mothers thought they should be accomplished. They also thought that the child should be able to walk a little sooner than the control group mothers did.

In general the fathers showed the same trend, particularly with regard to toilet training, but the differences between the two groups of fathers were less pronounced. It seems especially important that the standards of speech development expressed by the stuttering group fathers were considerably lower than those of their wives.

The fact that a mother has high standards of development for her child is likely to mean that even though the child is getting along normally the mother will not be wholly satisfied. He may be talking as fluently as the neighbor's children, but the mother may, even so, take his hesitations and repetitions to mean that his speech is below par and that he is beginning to "stutter."

In all my years of counseling parents who have been concerned about their children's speech, the one thing about them that has impressed me most has been their general degree of perfectionism. They differ among themselves, of course; some are very fussy and hard to please, others less so, but in general they have appeared, as a group, to be inclined to demand a little more of their children in the way of growth and development than would seem to be realistic. As a consequence, the problem does not always lie in what the child does, but rather in how far this falls short of what his parents think he should do.

◆ ◆ ◆

In this general vein, what are your own feelings about your children? Do you like them just the way they are, or do you wish they were different in some way?

We found that a few more of the stuttering than control group mothers said they wished their children were more alert. Another interesting difference was that roughly a third of the stuttering group mothers, nearly twice as many as in the control group, indicated that they wished their children would be either less or more cautious — and, moreover, they were about evenly divided between those who wished the child would be less and those who wished he would be

95

more cautious. More of the control group mothers said they would like their children to stay just as they were in this respect.

About the same numbers of parents in the two groups expressed a desire to have their children be more or less mischievous, cooperative, aggressive, self-confident, popular, or well mannered. Moreover, the two groups of parents expressed about the same degree of satisfaction with the intelligence of their children. It is interesting that there were relatively few parents in either group who said they wanted their children to be more attractive.

On a great majority of such ratings the two groups of parents were about alike. Such differences as there were, however, indicated higher standards, or greater dissatisfaction, on the part of the parents in the clinical group.

◄ ◄ ◄

To spank or not to spank, to be strict or easygoing — how do you feel about these basic questions of discipline?

It seemed that our stuttering group parents were a bit less satisfied with the way they were handling the discipline of their children. More control than stuttering group mothers felt that their children were well behaved. Also, more control group mothers felt that their husbands were "about right" rather than too strict or too lax in dealing with the children. More clinical than control group mothers said they were bothered "a great deal" when the child "made a mess around the house."

When asked how frequently their children were punished, the two groups of fathers gave about the same answers, but the stuttering group mothers reported more frequent punishment than did the mothers in the control group. It is extremely interesting, therefore, that when the parents were asked whether or not their children were punished for each of eighteen specific activities, their answers showed that on the average it was the control group children who were punished for the greater number of these activities. Of the eighteen activities, those for which punishment was most often reported were "talking back," "disobedience," "being noisy," "fighting with other children," "being rude," and "destroying things."

So far as differences with respect to particular misbehaviors were concerned, more control group parents said their children were "punished regularly for quarreling with other children," and for "talking back." There were no group differences, however, in the frequency with which the children were punished for messing up their own rooms, for spilling, disobedience, interrupting conversation, lying, swearing, fighting with other children, being rude, destroying things, and getting dirty.

The methods of punishment used were nearly the same for both groups. Spanking, the method most commonly used, was reported by roughly 40 per cent of the parents in both groups. Other methods, reported by 10 per cent or so of the parents, were taking privileges away, having the child sit on a chair, and sending the youngster to his room.

◀   ◀   ◀

Possibly you share the general idea that stuttering in children reflects tension in the home. This notion is widely held, though perhaps nearly always in the form of a vague hunch.

We succeeded in gathering some information that was related to this general theory. By carrying out a rather elaborate analysis of much of our data, we were able to gauge how much the mothers and fathers agreed and disagreed in various ways. Moreover, on some interview items we were able to make (a) a comparison of the mothers' and fathers' self-ratings, (b) a comparison of the mothers' and fathers' ratings of each other, (c) a comparison of the mother's rating of herself and the father's rating of the mother, and finally (d) a comparison of the father's rating of himself and the mother's rating of the father. The kinds and amounts of disagreement between the mothers and fathers — that is, specific pairs of husbands and wives — revealed by means of this analysis gave some indication of the "tension in the home" for the two groups of families.

The interview items on which husbands and wives disagreed were about equally divided between the two groups. For example, the husbands in both groups rated their own employment as more challenging than it was rated by their wives. Both groups of husbands had had a little more education than their wives. The husbands belonged to more organizations. It is especially interesting that the

97

husbands rated the appearance of their wives better than it was rated by the wives themselves.

The wives confided in their husbands more than the husbands confided in their wives. According to self-ratings the wives were more tense than their husbands were, and the husbands were more easygoing than their wives were. The husbands rated their wives as more irritable than the wives rated their husbands. The wives rated their own standards of conduct higher than they were rated by their husbands.

Here are a couple that are a little complicated: The wives said their husbands were away from home more than the husbands said their wives were away from home; and the husbands more often thought their wives were with the children too much than the wives thought their husbands were with the children too much.

The husbands apparently had more physical energy than their wives, according to both self-ratings and the ratings the husbands and wives made of each other. More husbands than wives said they had never studied or thought about child development norms, and the wives compared their children with the norms more frequently than their husbands did.

More wives than husbands were teetotalers.

Finally, the mothers were more annoyed or irritated by their children than the fathers were—and, incidentally, the interviewers gained the impression that the mothers talked more than the fathers did during the interviews.

It is especially interesting to see how the fathers and mothers disagreed with each other when the disagreement was found in one group of parents and not in the other. Here are some of the significant differences between the parents—between pairs of husbands and wives, that is—in the stuttering group. (These differences were not found in the control group.) They indicate that, in general, the fathers felt a little better about their children than the mothers did. They seemed to accept themselves more fully too. And they rated their wives for the most part a bit more favorably than they were rated by their wives.

The stuttering group fathers said the children played with other children better than the mothers said they did. More mothers than fathers said the following: the children gave up easily on hard tasks, the children felt picked on, the children had strong fears (other than any fears they may have had — or were thought to have — about speech). More mothers than fathers, however, said the children were not jealous.

The stuttering group fathers thought their wives felt more pride in their own accomplishments than their wives said they felt; and more mothers than fathers rated themselves unfavorably with respect to pride in their own accomplishments. The fathers rated their wives' standards of conduct higher than the mothers rated their husbands' standards of conduct. The mothers rated themselves as more tense than their husbands rated them. The mothers worried more about their health than the fathers worried about theirs. All these differences were found in the clinical, but not in the control, group.

Here are some additional similar items: More fathers said no than mothers predicted would say no in response to "As a general rule, do you feel a child should be seen and not heard?" The mothers did not say the children responded to suggestions or corrections as well as their husbands thought they would. The fathers rated their children more favorably than their wives thought they would in respect to "how well the child meets ideal standards." The fathers enjoyed having the child's friends come to the home more than their wives thought they did.

It is also of interest that the fathers rated the children's intelligence more favorably, in comparison with that of the neighbor children, than did the mothers, and more of them said the children were well behaved. More fathers than mothers thought that the spouse worried too much and was too demanding of the child.

Some of the more important differences between the clinical group husbands and wives had to do with their feelings about the child's speech. For example, more mothers than fathers said they thought about their child's speech while lying in bed at night, and that they talked to neighbors and relatives about it. More fathers than mothers said they did not accept the idea at first that the child was "stuttering." More fathers than mothers said that as far as they knew the child had never avoided any speaking situations. More mothers than fathers said they thought the child had especially difficult periods in speech. More mothers than fathers said the child was punished for "talking back."

More of the mothers than of the fathers said they were concerned about the child's speech when they first thought there was anything wrong with it, and in general more mothers than fathers reacted in one way or another to whatever it was they took to be the child's stuttering.

The two groups differed in the way the husbands and wives shared their discontent, and this was probably one of the most important differences between the two groups of parents. In the control group the discontent that was expressed appeared to be more or less equally shared by the mothers and fathers. The overall picture of disagreement within the stuttering group was, by contrast, one of somewhat more dissatisfaction on the part of the mothers. In fact, if the sharing was not wholly equal in the control group it was the fathers who were the less serene; when there was tension or disagreement, it indicated in half or more of the cases a conflict between a relatively contented mother and a somewhat discontented father. In the stuttering group, on the other hand, the disagreements that were found usually involved a conflict between a relatively contented father and a discontented mother.

The temptation is strong to conclude, therefore, that it is better, or less bad, for a child to have a somewhat unserene father, or even two parents who are companions in discontent, than it is for him to have a disenchanted mother — if he must be offered one or another of these somewhat dismal choices.

Many of the differences we found were probably due to the fact that the father had more freedom to come and go and to get away from the home, and that the mother was with the child much more of the time than the father was. The father was not generally as concerned about the child as the mother was, and so he was less concerned about the child's speech. At any rate, there were differences between the mothers and fathers, and some of these differences amounted to disagreements, or made disagreement more likely. In this sense, they represented "tension in the home." The more tension of this kind there is in a home, the more likely is a child to be caught up in the effects of parental differences and disagreements. One possible result of this can be that someone, more often than not the mother, finds his speech to be a source of dissatisfaction and concern, along with all the other things about which there is a lack of concord and contentment. "Tension in the home" is one of the things that parents who feel their child is stuttering should think about, at least a little.

◆　◆　◆

If you feel that your child is stuttering, it is practically a foregone conclusion that you are worried. In that case you are like the parents in our clinical group. They showed greater concern, worry, and sensitivity about their children's speech than the parents in the control group felt about the speech of their youngsters. Nearly 10 per cent of the clinical group parents said they even felt some degree of shame over their children's speech.

It is to be considered, of course, that we sampled the attitudes of the two groups of parents, not before the problem of stuttering arose, but eighteen months later than that, on the average. The clinical group parents started worrying about their children's speech, however, before their children did, and while their children were talking essentially the way the control group children were talking, as far as we could determine. However, once they began to worry they set in motion a vicious cycle in which the more bothered they became the more they bothered the child, and the more bothered the child became the more he bothered the parents, and so on and on. By the time we arrived on the scene the clinical group parents were very probably more concerned about their children's speech than they had been originally — but it seems clear that one of the reasons they were was that they had decided in the first place that what their youngsters were doing was "stuttering." It is important in this connection that more control than stuttering group parents indicated that they accepted repetitions and hesitations as part of "normal speech."

101

In view of the fact that the clinical group parents were as worried as they seemed to be, it is strange and doubtless significant that almost none of them had done much reading about stuttering. Roughly 95 per cent of both our groups reported that they had not read at all or slightly at most. In fact, seven out of ten had done no reading whatever about the problem.

Why had they not sought out books, pamphlets, and magazine articles in order to inform themselves as best they could? The easy answer is, of course, that we do not read much on any subject. People in the United States do not read as much as do people in England, the Scandinavian countries, and certain other parts of the world. This explains little or nothing, however, and needs itself to be explained. Besides, the parents we interviewed probably had read less about the stuttering problem than about many other subjects. This was to be expected undoubtedly of the control group. But why had so few in the clinical group read about stuttering?

An interesting possible answer to this question is that, although they were concerned about their children's speech, they were not concerned enough to go to the trouble of trying to inform themselves about the problem through reading. Now, one reason they may not have been sufficiently concerned was that, perhaps in most cases, the parents really felt that there was not very much the matter with the child's speech. In other words, they were worried but what they were worried about did not seem, even to them, to be enough to justify a visit to the public library. This fits well with what we know about the speech of the children who were looked upon as stutterers by their parents. At least at first it must not have seemed to be particularly different from the speech of other children.

Another possible explanation is that, like most of us, the clinical group parents had been influenced all their lives in numerous ways to take for granted that the thing to do when you feel you have a problem is not to try to understand it and handle it yourself, but to find an expert or specialist and turn it over to him. So why read?

Still another explanation is that some, or even much, of what there was to read about the stuttering problem was either dull or confusing — or demoralizing. The hitch is that even if this were the case, those who had never read anything at all would never have found it out. It could, of course, help to account for the fact that most of those who had read something had not read very much.

Whether our explanations are sound or mistaken, the important fact remains that very few of the parents had done any reading to speak of about the stuttering problem. Perhaps this book may play some small part in helping to change this situation. At least, you who are reading these lines are doing your bit to swell the number of parents who may from this time forward say that they have read more than a very little about the problem called stuttering.

CHAPTER 7

How the Problem Begins

WHO first decided your child was beginning to stutter? And exactly when did someone first get this idea? There could hardly be any more important questions than these for you to try to answer — as accurately as you possibly can. Reading the answers given to the same questions by the hundreds of other parents in our research program will help you to appreciate the importance of these questions, and to answer them for yourself as fully and precisely as possible.

We asked each mother and father nearly 200 questions about the child's speech development and the beginnings of the problem that they had called stuttering. In each case the mother and father were interviewed separately, of course, and all the questions concerning speech development were asked of the parents in the control group as well as those in the stuttering group.

There were many questions which referred to the behavior that the parents had called stuttering, and we asked these questions also of as many of the control group parents as we could. This needs to be explained a bit.

We asked the parents who regarded their children as stutterers to tell us as exactly as they could, and even to demonstrate by means of imitation, just how their children had been speaking when they first thought they were beginning to stutter. The answers we got can be fairly well summarized by saying that for the most part the children had been repeating the first parts of words li li li like this, or whole words like like like this, or phrases, such as such as this; or the children had been hesitating, pausing, and interjecting sounds as anyone does who is uncertain of what to say next, sounds or words such as ah, well, er, uh.

What we did then was to ask the control group parents whether their children had ever done these things.

We discovered that, with respect to patterns of perception, there are evidently three kinds of parents. By that I mean that about half of the control group parents said that their children had never done such things as we described. As was stated much earlier in this book, however, we know that all children, from the first year of life on through childhood — and to some degree all adults — repeat sounds, words, and phrases and hesitate in various other ways in speaking. The parents in the control group who said their children never did these things were evidently saying, in effect, that they had never perceived or noticed their children doing these things. They were telling us, therefore, something very important about the way they listened to their children. They apparently had been paying much more attention to their children's ideas, to the things they said, than to the way they sounded when they said these things.

The rest of the control group parents, a bit more than half, said that their children had spoken with repetitions and hesitations and they added, in effect, "Don't all children?" They regarded such disfluencies in speech as normal and made no issue of them.

Finally, of course, there were the parents in our clinical group who had all noticed their children repeating and hesitating, and had regarded their disfluencies as unusual or abnormal, and had classified them as "stuttering."

Now, as I have said, we asked the parents in the clinical group a very considerable number of questions about what they referred to as their children's stuttering. We asked these same questions of those control group parents who had said that their children spoke with hesitations and repetitions. In questioning the control group parents, however, we talked about repetitions and hesitations rather than "stuttering."

◆   ◆   ◆

How old was your child when he first began to stutter?
We put this seemingly simple question to all the mothers and

105

fathers in the clinical group. We put the same question to the parents in the control group this way: "How old was the child when you began to notice his speech in these respects?" (By "in these respects" we meant, of course, the hesitations and repetitions which these parents had said they had noticed in their children's speech, but had not thought of as "stuttering.")

We learned that the answer you get depends, first of all, upon who gives you the answer. To take our clinical group first, the answers we obtained from the mothers were different from those we got from the fathers. The average mother and father (pair of parents) in the clinical group gave answers that differed by five and one-half months! And in the average case what they were trying to recall had happened only eighteen months before. It seems reasonable to suppose that if any very definite, or clean-cut, or extremely grave change had come over the child's speech, the parents would have been able to agree better than they did on when it had happened. The fact that the mothers and fathers, pair by pair, disagreed as much as they did — by nearly a half-year — suggests that probably the beginning of the problem was not a clearly defined event of the sort that would register sharply in the parents' memory.

Then, just what was the beginning of the problem like? What was it like in your case?

Interestingly enough, one important approach to this question was to ask the control group parents how old their children were when they had begun to notice that the children were speaking with hesitations and repetitions. Half or more of the control group children were said to have begun to speak with such disfluencies when they were about three years old.

It is curious that their parents said they *began* to speak with repetitions and hesitations at that time. We know they do not *begin* to do these things when they are three years old. The fact is that they do them a little more frequently when they are two than when they are three. What the parents in both groups must have been reporting, without realizing it, was not mainly that their children had started speaking differently at a certain age, but rather that they, the parents, had started listening to them differently.

One of the facts that points to this conclusion is that the mothers and fathers, taken pair by pair, disagreed so greatly about the age at which the child began, as they said, to stutter — or, in the case of the control group parents, to speak with hesitations and repetitions. We have already noted the disagreement in these reports on the part of the parents in the clinical group; the parents in the control group disagreed even more wildly. In the average case in the control group the age given by the mother as that when the child had begun to speak disfluently differed from the age given by the father by 10.7 months, almost a full year! Had they been reporting a distinct and marked change that occurred in the speech of the child it seems hard to believe that they would have disagreed so greatly in reporting the time when it occurred. They might well have disagreed as much as they did, however, if they were reporting a change in their own ways of paying attention to the child when he was speaking. It would have been only by chance, of course, that changes in their personal listening habits would have occurred at precisely the same time.

There is another interesting fact to be noted in this connection. In Study II the children investigated were somewhat older than were those in Study III. In Study II the average age of the clinical group children was eight years and eight months and in Study III it was five years. Because the children were older in Study II the interval between the onset of the stuttering problem and the interview was longer than it was in Study III — a little over four years compared with eighteen months on the average. The effect of this longer interval on the memories of the mothers and fathers was apparently marked, because the mean difference between the mothers' and fathers' reports of the age when the stuttering problem began in Study II was a little over fifteen months, more than a full year. Moreover, the average child's age at the time when the problem of stuttering was reported to have begun was nearly four years according to the mothers in Study II, and three years and a half as reported by the mothers in Study III. The answer you get to the question of when stuttering begins depends, apparently, not only on who gives you the answer but also on when you ask the question — that is, how long after the event supposedly occurred.

107

The answer you get depends, too, on the way you ask the question. We not only asked the parents how old the child was when he had begun to stutter, but later on in the interview we also asked them how old the child was when they first felt that he had a speech problem. Suppose you stop and think about this in your own case. Did you think your child was stuttering and then sometime later decide he really had a problem, or did you think he had some sort of speech problem and after a while decide it was stuttering?

After the average mother in Study III had decided her child was beginning to stutter it took her nearly five months to come to the conclusion that he definitely had a speech problem. The main thing this seems to mean is that whatever the mother took to be stuttering, she did not consider it serious enough at first to regard it as a definite problem.

There seemed to be certain fairly definite reasons why the parents finally decided the child had a speech problem. One of these was that the time was approaching more and more closely when he would be entering school, and, while the parents had not taken the child's way of speaking very seriously before, they did regard it as a problem in connection with his entrance into school. Another kind of explanation is that in many, perhaps in most, cases the parents seemed to think of what the child was doing, which they had called stuttering, as a stage through which he would pass. They believed, or at least hoped, that he would "grow out of it." The fact that in the average case they decided after about five months that the child definitely had a speech problem would seem to indicate that for some reason they thought of "the stage through which the child would pass" as lasting about five months. When "the stage had not passed" within five months, they began to wonder whether it ever would pass. When they began to doubt that it would, they decided the child had a problem.

¶ ¶ ¶

These various considerations point to the general conclusion that whatever it was that the parents had noticed when they decided that "stuttering had begun" probably did not add up to any very striking change in the child's speech behavior. It is possible, of course, that there had been no change at all in the youngster's speech. The parents seemed to be reporting primarily their own dawning and growing — and wavering — feelings of uncertainty about the way the child was talking rather than any sudden and dramatic change in the child's speech itself.

Additional light is thrown on the matter by the answers we got when we asked the parents to "describe the situation in which the child stuttered the very first time." Now, one of the most important bits of information that we gained by asking this question was that only about 15 per cent of the parents claimed to be able to recall "the first situation in which the child stuttered." Do you feel sure that you can recall your child's very first instance of stuttering to the day and hour and the exact situation in which it occurred?

You will be interested to learn just what kinds of situations were described by the parents — by those, that is, who could report any. These are approximately the descriptions they gave of them: telling parents something; when he came in to tell something; reciting a piece at home; asking for something at the table; trying to get mother's attention; talking about what had happened while riding in a car after a slight accident and while competing with others for the privilege of speaking; asking the parents for something; telling something at the table; explaining something to the parents; competing with a sibling for the privilege of speaking; after a fall from a table; competing with adults for the privilege of speaking; upon meeting the father at the railway station after the father's two-week absence and with the mother present; talking to the parents; telling relatives something; talking to playmates; when on a ride with parents and friends; asking the parents a question in the car; after a scolding; and calling to the mother after witnessing a parental "fight."

The distinctive thing about these situations, as described, is that most of them seem to have been commonplace. This impression is reinforced by additional information that we obtained. The interviewers were told that in any case in which the parent could not recall "the very first situation," they were to ask for a description of "the first situation that the parent can recall, in which he or she can recall the child stuttering." In response to this alternative question, the situations recalled by the great majority of the parents were essentially like those listed above. In fact, many of them were described in almost exactly the same words. The only new ones which might have been more or less upsetting to the child, so far as we could judge, were "talking after being hit by another child" and "arguing with parent over something," each of which was reported for one child, but only by one of the parents in each case.

Not only did nearly all the situations reported seem ordinary, but they were also described in words that were not very precise. Most of them are not the kinds of words that are about specific times and places. This is consistent with the impression I have gained from repeated intensive clinical interviewing of parents, such as that presented in Chapter 2, that in the great majority of cases, whatever the child was doing when the parents first began to feel that he was stuttering, and wherever he was doing it, he was apparently not reacting to circumstances that were out of the ordinary. As a very general rule, he was not doing anything remarkable enough for the parents to remember it at all clearly.

These rather curious facts can be best understood if we keep in mind that it was nearly always a lay person, without training in speech pathology, who first decided that the child was stuttering. In only four instances in our largest research sample of 150 cases was the original judgment, or "suspicion," or "diagnosis" made by some kind of professionally trained person — in two cases by a teacher, in one by a physician, and in one by a school nurse. In not even one case was the original judgment, or diagnosis, made by a specialist in speech disorders. In roughly nine out of ten cases it was the parents themselves, usually the mother, who first decided the child was "stuttering." In nearly all the remaining cases the original decision was made by other members of the family, particularly grandparents.

Our findings in this connection may be summarized by saying that, as a general rule, the problem of stuttering seems to begin as a judgment made of the child's speech by some member of the child's family, practically always one or both of the parents, usually the mother. In the great majority of cases there is no apparent disagreement between the mother and father concerning this judgment, regardless of which one makes it first. Almost never do the parents check their own judgment against that of a professional speech pathologist. For several months, even years, in the usual case the parents rely entirely upon their own "diagnosis" of the child's speech. Even when they do eventually seek clinical help their purpose is not to have their "diagnosis" checked by experts, but rather to "have the stuttering cured" or at least to obtain advice about treatment or remedial instruction. It is, indeed, one of the most interesting and important facts about the problem called stuttering that it is, with very rare exceptions, diagnosed by laymen, and it is attended to at first, usually for several months or even for two or three years or longer, without benefit of professional consultation.

Has this been true in your case?

❧   ❧   ❧

In order to gain more information about the circumstances surrounding the onset of the problem we asked, in a long series of questions, whether each of several kinds of specific conditions was present in the first situation in which the child was thought to stutter, or the first situation the parents could recall, even though it was not the first situation in which they believed the child was stuttering.

The conditions most often said to be present in the situations recalled were these: hurry in speaking, excitement, difficulty in finding the right word, competing for the privilege of speaking, trying to "hold the floor," and speaking to an unresponsive listener (such as father behind a newspaper in the evening or mother busy fixing dinner). These would seem to be rather ordinary conditions. The more unusual and presumably more serious conditions, such as severe fright, shame, punishment, conflict involving disobedience, and changes in environment, were seldom reported. Conditions like frustration or bewilderment, illness or fatigue, and difficulty of the children in making themselves understood, reported by less than 10 per cent of the informants, may be thought of as lying between these two general classes of circumstances.

In asking these questions we were to some extent unavoidably "putting words in the parents' mouths." Instead of relying wholly upon the memories of the mothers and fathers, we were suggesting that certain conditions might have been present by the very act of asking whether they had, in fact, been present. Even so, the great majority of the parents gave "No" responses to all these items, except for "hurry in speaking."

There seems to be little room for doubt, on the basis of our data, that in the usual case the parents first get the idea that their children are beginning to stutter in situations that are decidedly commonplace. In describing these situations, the parents almost never tell about anything that sounds like a crisis.

◀   ◀   ◀

Has it occurred to you to wonder whether your child could have begun to stutter by imitating another child who was stuttering?

This view is more or less popular, and so the facts we have been able to gather in this connection are especially interesting. About one third of the children brought to us by their parents as stutterers were said to have been in close or frequent contact with one or more stutterers. Between 15 and 20 per cent of the parents said they felt that the speech of their children resembled that of other stutterers — but, curiously enough, only about 10 per cent of the children were said to know about the stuttering of these other stutterers, and it seems clear that they could not have imitated speech they did not know about. Moreover, of these, less than half, or under 5 per cent of all cases, had found out about the speech of the other stutterers by actually hearing them talk; the rest had evidently been told about it. Finally, although when asked, "What do you think caused your child's stuttering?" eight fathers and three mothers, out of a total of 300 parents, gave "imitation" as one answer, actually in another part of the interview no mother or father included the child's imitation of stuttering among the conditions or circumstances associated with the beginning of the problem.

Anyone who has watched television or stage performers who are good at doing imitations realizes that an acceptable imitation of a moderate or severe stutterer, or even a mild one, requires considerable skill. It is not clear, therefore, precisely what the few parents who used the term "imitation" meant by it. At any rate, it does seem clear that imitation, however defined, is of very slight, if any, importance in relation to the onset of the stuttering problem.

◄   ◄   ◄

In summary, through our research and clinical studies we have found that as a rule parents remember only vaguely, if at all, the situations in which they first felt that their children were beginning to stutter. The onset of the problem is practically never reported as having occurred under dramatic or memorable circumstances. On the contrary, the relatively few parents who claim they can remember the situations in which they first thought their children were stuttering describe these situations nearly always as commonplace and unremarkable. The conditions they report most often are those of hurried speech and excitement, conditions under which most, if not all, young children usually speak with something less than perfect fluency. In fact, our control group parents also said that the most common conditions under which they first thought their children were speaking repetitiously and hesitantly were those of excitement and hurry. In other words, the conditions that were said to be associated with the "first stutterings" of the clinical group children were in general the same as those associated with the "first" hesitations and repetitions of children who were looked upon by their parents as normal speakers.

The findings from our research on the onset of the problem called stuttering, then, do not support the traditional notion that the problem begins as a rule when the child suddenly starts to have some sort of serious difficulty in speaking, under conditions of illness, great fright, injury, unusual emotional stress, or some other kind of crisis. On the contrary, when someone, usually one of the parents, first decides the child is beginning to stutter, he is not likely to be doing anything very unusual, nor is it probable that the circumstances are remarkable enough to be remembered later by his parents.

These facts are very hopeful. They indicate that parents who feel

113

that their children are stutterers have good grounds for believing that they are quite like other children who are regarded by their parents as normal speakers. If all I knew about your youngster was that you had decided that he had begun to stutter, my best guess would have to be that he is basically as normal as pumpkin pie in Kansas in November.

CHAPTER 8

How the Problem Develops

THE research we have done indicates that in the most representative case the problem of stuttering arises under quite ordinary circumstances. It arises when the child involved is between three and four years old, and at the moment when the child's mother begins to doubt that he is speaking all right. What sort of speaking is the child doing at this time and in these circumstances?

Though most parents say they can't recall the very first time they thought the child was stuttering, nearly all can give some account of the way the youngster was talking during the general period when they felt he was beginning to stutter. The accounts they give are much like those of the few parents who do claim to be describing the child's speech as it was the first time they looked upon him as a stutterer. In general, as we have already seen, in the most representative case the youngster, when his parents think he is starting to stutter, is repeating words, or the first sounds or syllables of words, or occasionally whole phrases, or he is hesitating by saying something like "uh uh uh." He is doing these things with no apparent awareness that he is doing them or that they are of any significance, and he is showing no notable tension or effort. Moreover, he is apparently doing these things only about as often or as much as most other children of his age do.

Now, are there exceptions to this "most representative case"? This is a very important question and you are almost sure to ask it. And you probably want to know what the exceptions, if there are any, are like and how they might best be explained. You may feel that your own child is an exception.

115

We have seen, in Chapter 2, an example of one kind of case that looks, at first, like an exception. You will recall that Mrs. Smith said that when her daughter Alice was about two and a half years old she began to speak repetitiously one Saturday morning. Her first repetition, Mrs. Smith said, was I I I I — and, to use Mrs. Smith's approximate words early in the interview, she continued from that time on to repeat every time she said anything. This sounds like a good deal more than the average amount of repetition for the general run of children. However, Alice was not repeating "every time she spoke" when she visited our speech clinic at the age of five. In fact, her speech was not very remarkable according to our observations. And, you will recall, Mrs. Smith, after doing the best job she could of remembering that crucial Saturday morning and the days and weeks following it, decided that Alice had not repeated "every time," or anything like every time, she spoke.

Like Mrs. Smith we don't always say exactly what we mean. Moreover, we are not always sure just what we do mean. One of the fundamental reasons for this is that *the way we remember events is influenced by the words we use in telling about them.* You are, indeed, as I have put it in the title of a book, "your most enchanted listener." Whenever we talk to other people we are ourselves affected, as a rule, more than they are by what we say to them.

So it was that after Mrs. Smith had told enough other people — had told herself enough times, that is — that Alice had started to stutter "overnight" and had continued "from that time on to stutter every time she said anything" it became not only her story, it was for all practical purposes her very memory. As the transcript of the interview indicates, she was genuinely surprised when she realized, while trying to reconstruct the sequence of events as carefully as she could, that no, it had not been "every time" after all, come to think of it. It is clear that she had no intention whatever of stretching or distorting the facts. It is also clear that she had managed to get them not quite straight. And how very much like you and me and everyone else Mrs. Smith was in doing what she did. It is simply that we preserve the past in our own words, and our own words do not always —

perhaps we should even say seldom — correspond closely to what actually happened.

Some of the apparent exceptions to our most representative case turn out, therefore, not to be exceptions.

Here is another example of this sort of apparent exception, as represented by a few lines taken from the transcript of a tape-recorded interview with the mother of a four-and-a-half-year-old boy. Names, as always, are disguised.

INTERVIEWER (I): Where — did someone else tell you that he had a speech problem, or did you think he had, or —

MRS. JONES (MJ): No one else told me. One day he just couldn't get words out for five minutes.

I: Oh, I see. Tell me about this. You must remember it pretty vividly, don't you?

MJ: No, not particularly. Just one day —

I: Well — five minutes is a long time.

MJ: Well, it is a long time.

I: And you think it was five minutes?

MJ: Well — I wouldn't want to be pinned down. It was, it was, but it — he wasn't repeating it just two or three times.

I: Would you please try now to repeat, to say "you" now over and over and repeat it until I tell you to stop? O.K., begin.

MJ: (Started repeating "you" and continued until signaled to stop.)

I: That was ten seconds. Do you think he did that sort of thing for five minutes?

MJ: (Laughter.) No, probably not . . .

I: Did he do it that long, ten seconds?

MJ: I think he could have.

I: Twice that long, or just that long?

MJ: No, I doubt if it would be twice that long.

I: So it would be something under twenty seconds then?

MJ: I really don't know. I never timed it.

I: So when you said five minutes (laughter by Mrs. Jones) this was a manner of speaking, was it? This was not information, then, but a sort of expression?

MJ: I'd say so . . .

◄ ◄ ◄

Sometimes, of course, it is impossible to establish just what did happen. Our memories are not always good enough. The parents cannot say just when the problem first arose and they cannot describe the first instance of it or say for sure what the child's speech was like at the time. We can't be absolutely sure whether such cases are exceptions to our most representative case, and yet the clearest indication is that they are not exceptions in any important sense, because they appear not to involve anything very much out of the ordinary. Here is a good example, taken from a tape-recorded interview of a mother and father:

INTERVIEWER (I): Could you tell me — when did it begin?

MRS. BROWN (MRS. B): Well, I suppose he's been doing it for about the last two years now.

I: What was the problem like when it began?

MRS. B: Well, he, uh, at first he didn't stutter all the time, just at certain times. Then maybe he'd do it for a month and then maybe he would quit for a while.

I: I see. And when he did it, right at first — can you remember by any chance the first day?

MRS. B: No.

I: Can you, Mr. Brown?

MR. B: No, I can't.

I: Can you remember pretty near the first day? (Pause.) You can't tie it down to any event?

MRS. B: I can't tie it down to any — (pause)

I: It wasn't just before Christmas, or just after the Fourth of July, or just before the big blow, or the big flood, or there wasn't a fire on the neighbor's farm that you remember things by?

MRS. B: No, I don't — not any incident that I can remember.

I: You hadn't just taken a trip?

MRS. B: Of course, right at the time you don't try and remember. You know, you don't think too much about it then, I mean, its continuing.

I: Yes, I realize that. But there was no illness, injury, nothing that stood out?

MR. B: Well, that time he hit his head.

MRS. B: Yes, but — I don't — did he stutter before that?

I: When did he hit his head? I'm just trying to get a date. I don't want to —

MRS. B: Well, that was in the summer of — it would be two years ago, wouldn't it?

MR. B: Three years.

MRS. B: Three?

I: You think three and you think two?

MR. B: It has to be three years ago.

MRS. B: We didn't go this year, we didn't go last year, we went the year before.

I: That would be two years ago. Where did you go?

MRS. B: We went to a picnic and it was like a — where the kids played it was a bandstand and there used to be an old wading pool there and he fell down —

I: Oh, I see.

MRS. B: He fell down off that.

I: I see. Was he badly hurt?

MRS. B: A light concussion.

I: A light concussion. Well, in terms of what you did with him, did he have to go to a hospital, or —?

MRS. B: Well, we took him over to Watertown and they X-rayed him and they said there was a slight crack back in here from a concussion there. His eye was all black and — looked like the blood had all run down there.

I: He went to bed for a few days?

MRS. B: Well, they said — it was funny — they told me they couldn't find anything and they said, "Why, he'll be all right, just take him home."

I: So he was up and about then?

MRS. B: Oh yes, he was up and around.

I: Now, can you tell me how he was talking just before the picnic?

MRS. B: Well, I don't believe he stuttered too much because he, when he first started to talk he talked just as plain, just as plain as could be.

I: And after the picnic, you don't remember — or do you remember?

MRS. B: Well, I don't remember that he started right at that time. He must have gradually worked into it then.

I: Well, I don't want to relate these events unless they were related.

MRS. B: Well, I, uh, I really — (pause)

I: What time of the year was this?

MRS. B: That was in the summertime.

MR. B: August, wasn't it? Around the first of August?

MRS. B: I think probably — that's when they always have it.

I: Umhm. And he's five now, he'd have been three then. Now, awhile ago you told me when he was around two you thought it started. Was that right, or did I misunderstand you?

MRS. B: Well, I suppose it was a little later than that —

119

I: I see. But do you remember — that is, can you now relate any observation you made about his speech to this incident? I don't want to blow up the incident. I'm trying to get a date on the calendar. This was early in August in 1954. Can you remember August of '54 so far as his talking is concerned?

MRS. B: I don't think he stuttered right then because right after — (pause)

I: All right. Then you can't remember the beginnings of this problem?

MRS. B: Well, let's see, he would have been about three then — (pause)

I: Yes?

MRS. B: I think he must have been about three and a half.

I: Sometime in the winter, then? But you can't pinpoint it to a day?

MRS. B: I can't say for sure because I never wrote it down and I didn't think anything about it.

I: Yes — and so, am I to conclude from this then that when it started it didn't amount to much?

MRS. B: No, it really didn't.

I: Do you also agree to this, Mr. Brown?

MR. B: Yes . . .

I: It didn't amount to much. What was it like? Can you remember?

MRS. B: Well, he just stuttered on the first —

I: I know, but how did he do this? How did it sound? Can you imitate it? Now don't answer unless you can remember, but if you can remember what you first noticed that you worried about, or noticed as though it were worth noticing, whether you worried or not — what was this?

MRS. B: I can't remember.

I: Can you remember, Mr. Brown?

MR. B: No, I can't.

I: Umhm. All right. Can you tell me when you did first begin to notice something that you can remember?

MRS. B: Well, I think he stutters just mostly any word — I mean —

I: What I want to know is when, thinking back from now — this is November 1956 — when did you begin to feel that Mike had a speech problem that you should do something about — that you were worried about?

MRS. B: Oh, I suppose the last six months.

I: The last six months? So that would make it last April, around Easter? Now, what do you remember around Easter, then, in the way of a definite event or a time when you looked at him and you decided, "We've got to do something about this," or, "There's something the matter here" — whatever you thought? Can you tell me when that was? You don't remember the day? Or the event, or the occasion?

MRS. B: No, I can't relate it to any certain — (voice trailed off)

The Browns are essentially like many other parents. What they said in effect summarizes many and many a case: The problem came on gradually, and they couldn't say just when it began. Parents who give this sort of account do not talk about a specific incident, or a precise moment of onset of the problem. They talk about a period of time that lasted from a few days perhaps to a year or more. During this time their feeling that the child was beginning to stutter grew gradually, with ups and downs, into a conviction. In Study III only 15 per cent, or about one out of six, of the parents claimed to be able to remember the first time they regarded the child as a stutterer — and even most of the few who said they could did not seem to have very clear memories of it.

Close examination of all the data we have collected strongly suggests that the major reason parental memories of the beginnings of the problem are so dim is that there is as a rule not much to be remembered.

This is well indicated by the fact that nearly nine out of ten of the clinical group children in Study III were said to have been repeating the first syllables of words, or whole words, or phrases when someone first decided they were stuttering. We know that such repetitions occur more or less frequently in the speech of all children, and indeed were the sorts of things most often reported in Study III by the control group parents who said they had noticed disfluencies in the speech of their children.

The differences and similarities between the two groups of children in this connection were most interesting. Syllable repetitions (su su such as this) were reported for a significantly larger proportion of the clinical group children, but repetitions of phrases (such as this, such as this) were reported for a significantly larger proportion of the control group children, and there was no appreciable difference between the two groups in word repetition (such such such

121

as this). More of the clinical group children were said to have prolonged the first sounds of words, and more of the control group youngsters hesitated by pausing and saying "uh uh uh" and the like. By and large, when the clinical group children were first considered by their parents to be starting to stutter they were evidently speaking about the way the control group youngsters were when their parents began to take note of the fact that they did not always speak fluently.

❦   ❦   ❦

But were there not exceptions? The common view seems to be that more or less suddenly one day stuttering begins in the form of a tense speech block of some sort. We took special pains, therefore, to determine in each case whether the child had been speaking with noticeable tension, or having what might be called a severe speech block, or suffering an "inability to get the word out" when he was first thought to be stuttering.

We asked the parents in the clinical group this question: At the time when stuttering was first noticed, was the child using force or more effort than usual "to get his words out"? Was there more than usual muscular tension? We put the same question to those parents in the control group who said their children had spoken with hesitations and repetitions, except that for them we did not use the word "stuttering." The two groups of parents gave answers that were remarkably similar. About a third of the mothers in the clinical group answered yes to this question — but so did one out of every five of those in the control group. Most of the stuttering group mothers who reported tension said it was slight.

We also asked these five questions: Did the child seem indifferent to his very first stoppages? When the stuttering was first noticed did the child seem to be aware of the fact that he was speaking in a different manner or doing something wrong? Did the child show surprise or bewilderment after having had trouble on a word? Did the very first stoppages seem to be unpleasant to the child? Do you think the child felt irritated when the very first stoppages occurred?

Roughly nine out of ten of the parents in both groups indicated

122

that the children seemed oblivious or indifferent to what they were doing and showed no emotionality about it.

In my series of tape-recorded research interviews I have not yet had a parent tell me that the stuttering began with a tense blockage or anything of that sort. In Study III, however, we found nine out of 300 parents whose responses seemed to indicate that they had observed some kind of block or breakdown in speech as the first evidence of the stuttering problem. The reports of these nine mothers and fathers may be summarized in these words: (1) complete block on the first sound of a word; (2) repetition of a whole word and of the first syllable or sound of a word; complete block on the first sound of a word; (3) repetition of a word; block on the initial sound of a word; (4) block before a word, with gutteral sounds; (5) repetition of the first syllable of a word; block on the initial sound of a word; (6) repetition of the first sound or syllable of a word; complete block on the first sound of a word; prolongation of the initial vowel or consonant of a word; (7) repetition of a whole word, or of the first sound or syllable of a word; complete block on the first sound of a word; prolongation of the first consonant of word; interjection of "uh uh"; (8) repeated gasps; (9) block before a word.

Now, if such reports are to be taken at face value they suggest the possibility at least that in each case there had been some kind of striking, even alarming, difficulty. In view of this possibility, it seems very significant that whatever was meant by these words, it was reported, in every one of the nine cases, by only the father or the mother, never by both. If the parents were using such words seriously and thoughtfully they would have been talking about something different from ordinary speech behavior, possibly something sufficiently serious to disturb any parent observing it. It is not easy to see, therefore, why one of the parents in every case had somehow failed to observe this presumably extraordinary behavior, or at least could not remember having been told about it by the other parent who had apparently observed it.

In light of all the data, including the intensive research interviews, I am inclined to believe that the most likely explanation is that the nine mothers and fathers who made these reports did not use the words quoted as descriptive terms in the ordinary sense. The word "block," for example, as used in this connection, even by speech pathologists, does not seem as a rule to have a clear and definite meaning. It is not certain what the nine parents were referring to when they used it, especially in the expression "complete block."

Nevertheless, I think it is likely that the nine parents were trying to tell us about something that they had observed their children doing which in their judgment was important. I should prefer to regard these, for present purposes, as exceptions to our "most representative case." At any rate, I think there are exceptions to it and that it is important to account for them.

One explanation of apparent exceptions is the one we have already considered, that we don't always say quite what we mean — we say "every time" when we mean "once in a while" or "five minutes" when we mean "a few seconds." In the same vein, we undoubtedly sometimes say that a child had a "complete block" when we mean something much less dramatic or serious. In other words, what there is to be explained is what there is left after our ways of saying things sometimes have been properly discounted.

That still leaves some things to be explained, in my opinion. One explanation to be noted and put to one side is that children do a good deal of playing with the sounds they discover they can make. They try to sound like geese and chickens, and trains and tugboats — and they make a lot of sounds that are seemingly quite original. In experimenting with sound-making they sometimes tense up their mouths and throats and twist their tongues and huff and puff and generate a good deal of tension. Sometimes they do these things when they are talking — or instead of getting on with the talking their parents think they should be doing. We don't know as much about the vocal play of young children as we should, but on the basis of what we do know I think some of the things that parents occasionally refer to as "difficulty" or even "complete blocks" in speaking turn out, on a closer look, to be a kind of unusual playfulness, or vocal experimenting and exploring.

What is rather more important, in my judgment, is that there are many conditions under which young children — as well as older children and adults — speak with tension, excessive hesitation, and indeed in ways that give the appearance of "complete stoppage." In fact, I think that moderate to severe blockages in speech are sufficiently common that we might well expect more of them to be reported by parents in describing what they remember as their children's first stutterings. It is as necessary to explain the large majority of cases in which no such blockages are reported among the "first stutterings" as it is to account for the small minority in which they are. And the best explanation I can draw from our data is that parents, provided they notice the disfluencies in their children's speech and take them seriously, are most likely to regard them as stuttering *if they can see no reason for them.*

To me, this is one of the most surprising and fascinating conclusions that our data suggest. You see, our dictionaries, our speech authorities, and just about everyone else define "stuttering" as a disturbance in the rhythm or fluency of speech, marked by repetitions and hesitations, associated in some instances at least with tension or strain. It is a curious fact that although this definition is so widely taken for granted, it is also all but universally ignored or disregarded in certain cases.

For example, most persons who have cerebral palsy speak in a labored and disfluent manner, and yet their way of speaking is very seldom classified as stuttering. In many cases of aphasia, a form of disturbed speech and language resulting from some types of brain damage, the speech is halting, repetitious, and at times characterized by considerable tension, but it is practically never diagnosed as stuttering. We are all thoroughly familiar with the unsteady, hesitant, unrhythmical speech, marked at times by at least slight tension, of persons who are intoxicated, or drugged, or grief-stricken, or extremely fatigued, or deeply discouraged or depressed. We know, too, the disturbed speech of children and adults who are highly excited, or extremely angry, or greatly embarrassed or afraid. Almost never do we classify the speech observed under any of these conditions as stuttering. Why don't we, since it fits the generally accepted definition of "stuttering"?

I think the reason we don't is that whenever we can see what looks to us like a reason for speech to be disturbed we take for granted that there is nothing wrong *with the speech itself*. If your child has just been scared stiff by a terrific crash of thunder and is incoherent with tension in gasping repeated fragments of words, you are not likely to think he is stuttering — it is obvious to you that he is unable to talk better because he is scared. Or, if a youngster whose speech muscles are tense and incoordinated because of cerebral palsy says "Please pass the butter" hesitantly and laboriously, prolonging the first sound of "the," his mother is not going to decide he is stuttering, because she assumes that with cerebral palsy it is normal for him to talk that way.

Now, it is precisely under such conditions that children are most likely to exhibit anything very unusual in the way of tension or excessively disfluent or blocked speech. And since the disturbed speaking they do under such conditions is not likely to be thought of by their parents as stuttering, it follows that the beginnings of stuttering are not usually described as severe disturbances in speech fluency.

On the contrary, parents are most likely to decide their children are stuttering when they are hesitating and repeating *for no reason that the parents can detect*. And these are precisely the hesitations and repetitions that are not associated with anything obvious like great fright, excessive fatigue, great mortification, muscular paralysis, or incoordination. "No reason" can be any one of the reasons that the parents do not recognize or understand.

What reasons might these be? There are probably two major kinds. Under one may be grouped all the things that make children generally repeat and hesitate as much as they do when speaking under ordinary conditions. There are many such factors, some inborn, some learned, and some that are environmental in a passing or at least unremarkable sense. The human brain just doesn't work perfectly in transforming experience into spoken words. And some normal brains perform this amazing function less smoothly than other brains do — for reasons about which no one really knows very much. Moreover, any young child still has a lot to learn about using the language, and some children have more to learn than others.

The other reason children speak disfluently — the other reason, that is, that parents usually don't notice — is traceable to anything and everything that the parents themselves do that make a child doubt that he can speak well or smoothly enough to be accepted and approved by them, and that makes him feel concerned or uneasy about not being able to speak that well.

Most mothers and fathers have not been sufficiently prepared while in school, or by any other means, to recognize or understand very well either of these reasons for a child's disfluent speech.

Whenever the child repeats and hesitates for these reasons, then, to his parents he is doing so "for no reason" and, since they can see nothing wrong with anything else, they are likely to conclude that there must be something wrong *with his speech.* They are likely to do this, of course, only if they happen to notice the disfluency in the first place and give it a second troubled thought.

So it is that parents usually say that when they first felt their child was stuttering he was repeating words or the first parts of words, or hesitating by saying things like "uh uh uh," with no apparent tension or awareness, in circumstances that were not particularly remarkable in any way. The few who report some kind of more severe speech block are probably referring to speech disturbances associated with great fright, bewilderment, shame, fatigue, or the like. In some cases they actually refer to such factors. When they do not refer to them, a rather simple explanation is that they had not been aware of them because they were paying attention only to the child's disrupted speech, and they didn't notice the unusual conditions responsible for it.

The conditions that parents most often associate with either the first or early instances of what they have thought of as stuttering are hurry in speaking and excitement. These frequently seem to be one and the same thing, of course. In our research the control group parents also mentioned these as conditions under which their normally speaking children were disfluent in speech, and it is common knowledge, of course, that adults as well as children stumble in speaking, and run their words together and repeat, and in general speak less smoothly when excited or in a great hurry. In such a case a child might very well seem to be repeating excessively, or "having a great deal of trouble," even to be "blocked" or "unable to say a thing" — provided the parent disregards the excitement and the reasons for it. Now, in some instances the parents do fail to appreciate the excitement itself, and notice only the apparent breakdown in the child's speech, for the good reason that what the child is excited about is just not exciting at all to his parents. They are not even conscious of it. They focus their attention entirely on the disrupted way the youngster is talking and, seeing "no reason" for it, they are likely to jump to the disturbing conclusion that something is the matter with the child's speech itself.

◄   ◄   ◄

One of the most crucial facts in connection with this matter is the age at which the child is most likely to be first regarded as a stutterer. Our investigations have shown that very few parents report the onset of stuttering before the age of two and a half years. The average age falls between three and three and a half, and in the large majority of cases the onset occurs before the age of four years. About the only time it is said to occur after that is when the child enters school, and whenever this is the case it is practically always a teacher who first decides that the child is beginning to stutter, even though no one else has thought so up to that time.

Parents are pleased with their child's speech so long as they think that he is *learning* to talk. So long as they are listening for the signs of learning and development, they do not focus on imperfections. What they notice is that he is saying new words that he has never said before, that he is making longer and longer sentences, asking more and more questions, speaking to more and more people, and making more and more sense in one way or another. Then there comes a time, usually around the child's third birthday, when their attitude gradually changes because it becomes harder and harder for them to notice whether any learning is going on. By the time the youngster is three or so his vocabulary has become so large that it is not easy to tell when he has used a new word, none of his sentences stand out anymore as being a great deal longer than the longest ones he has previously uttered, he has already talked to every-body in the neighborhood, and in general he is talking so much that now, as far as the parents are concerned, he is no longer *learning* to speak. He has learned.

The youngster is now a speaker — and so the parents begin to judge him as a speaker. It is at this point, then, that they may notice that he repeats and hesitates. They had not previously noticed his repetitions and hesitations, and so they can say in all honesty that so far as they know he had never done these things before. They take for granted, therefore, that he is *beginning* to do them. If they think that children who are normal speakers do not repeat and hesitate, they conclude that their tike is not speaking normally. And if they can see no reason for his repeating and hesitating — and if they have the necessary motivations for doing so — they call what he is doing "stuttering." Actually, he was doing more repeating and hesitating six months previously, and even more six months before that, but then either the parents didn't notice his disfluencies at all, or else they accepted them as all right, or as "nothing," because they were more or less aware of a reason for them. The reason, which they took for granted, was that he was then too young to talk any better. For a little fellow of one and a half, or two, or two and a half, he was doing just fine, his parents thought, no matter how he was talking, because what they noticed above all else was that month by month, or week by week, even day by day he was talking better and better, and this pleased and delighted them.

◢ ◢ ◢

The parents' decision, then, that the child is beginning to "stutter" is one thing; the ways in which the child actually talks, in the mean-time, is something else again. There may be some relationship be-tween these two, and there may not be. It depends not only on what the youngster does when he talks, but also on the circumstances in which he does it, and precisely what his parents are paying atten-tion to while he is talking. Some parents pay attention to the circum-stances and think nothing of the child's repetitions and hesitations; others pay attention to the hesitations and repetitions and ignore the circumstances; and some don't pay much attention to either one. Moreover, some parents worry about the circumstances and some don't; others worry about the child's speech and others don't; and the rest see nothing to worry about in either the child's speech or the circumstances in which he speaks.

Parents differ in these ways because they bring differences in background and temperament and outlook to the situations in which they observe their children speaking. This means, of course, that in order to understand the problem called stuttering in your own specific case you must know as much or more about yourself as about your child. You must also know, in general, more than you ordinarily would about what your youngster does when he talks, the circumstances in which he does it, and how you tend to react both to what your child does and to the circumstances.

If you are to solve the problem, or bring about changes for the better, there are three main things, accordingly, about which you may need to do something: the way your child talks, the conditions that seem to affect the way he talks, and your own reactions to the way he talks. You cannot do very much in a direct way about your child's speech — that is, you cannot move with his muscles or make sounds with his throat. You can do something, however, to improve the conditions under which your child talks. You can do most of all about your own reactions to your child's speech.

Your reactions depend largely on how well informed you are about the speech behavior of children generally and the kinds of conditions that affect it favorably and badly — and you can improve your information. In fact, you are doing so by reading this book. Your reactions depend, too, on how much you know about your own child's speech behavior, particularly as compared with that of other children, and the specific conditions that affect it one way or another — and you can become more observant of these things. Your reactions also depend upon whether you talk about your youngster's speech in words that are negative and exaggerated and emotional. That sort of language tends to make you and others attentive to every bobble in your child's speech, and inclined to classify it as "stuttering" even when most objective observers would not, and to feel generally bad about it. If, on the other hand, you talk about your youngster's speech in terms that are simply descriptive of what he does — he repeats words, for example, he says "uh uh" and the like — and that refer appropriately to the conditions he is responding to when he does these things, your feelings about his speech are likely to be matter-of-fact, and your reactions will probably not cause your child to feel that you are hard to talk to. In such a case, he will not be so likely to become uneasy and tense trying to speak to you, and so you will respond more approvingly.

This is all very hopeful, because it means that there is a great deal you can do that can be helpful. You do not have to depend on someone else to do everything for you. Indeed, no one else can.

CHAPTER 9

The Sad-Go-Round

ONCE you had decided that your child was beginning to stutter, what did you feel and what did you do?

If you are like the majority of parents I have known in the clinic and the laboratory, you began to worry more or less. You did not lie awake night after night and brood about the problem day in and day out, but you thought about it off and on. At first, you didn't think of it as a very serious problem, largely because you half expected and half hoped that what you took to be your child's stuttering would "go away." You told yourself that perhaps it was a phase through which he would pass.

All the while, if you did about what most other parents do, you were paying attention to your child's hesitancies and repetitions, and although your attention wavered you became a little more attentive week by week. As you now look back on it, it seemed "to come on gradually." Eventually you became convinced that "it" was not going to go away — that if "it" was a stage, it was not one through which your youngster was going to pass. You decided that he really had a speech problem, and when you arrived at that conclusion you settled down to worry more or less constantly. You began to wonder if something shouldn't be done about it. In fact, you began to do certain things about it yourself.

At first, you didn't do much directly. Mostly when you thought your child was "having difficulty" in saying something you looked away from him, or you looked worried, you stiffened ever so little, or stopped smiling, or became thoughtful, or started knitting a little faster, or maybe you said or did something to change the subject.

But you did these things mostly without realizing what you were doing. In fact, you didn't think of these reactions as anything that you did about your child's speech. Having forgotten that you had done such things, or never having been particularly aware of doing them, you later told a speech clinician perhaps that you had "done nothing" about your child's stuttering, and that you were sure he would have had no way of knowing how you felt about it.

It was a little later that you began to suggest to your child, gently and not very often, that he speak more slowly, or calm down a little, or stop and start over, or take it easy and think out what he was going to say. On an occasional day you said something like this to him as many as five or ten times, and then you might go for several days without talking about it, though whenever you felt he was stuttering you would do the other things like tensing up a little, or knitting a little faster, or turning away as though you had just remembered to check the oven.

As time went on you may have said something to him now and then about his speech mainly to reassure him, telling him, for example, that you thought he was speaking just fine, or that you were sure he would soon be talking just like anyone else. Occasionally, he might have overheard you talking about the problem with his father, or with his grandparents, or a neighbor or friend of the family. Unless you are exceptional you have never scolded your youngster for what you take to be his stuttering, and you have probably never told him that you wished he would talk better, or that you didn't like the way he talked, or that it made you nervous to hear him stutter, or to please get out what he had to say without taking so much time. Mostly you have kept your worries and your feelings to yourself, or you have expressed them indirectly by facial expression, tone of voice, and posture, or you have spoken to your child gently, suggesting that he take his time, or just relax a little, or stop and think and start over perhaps.

These are the ways you have reacted if you are like most other parents. Some parents react in other ways, of course. Those who try to do anything about the child's breathing, such as telling him to take a deep breath before speaking, seem most likely to reap unfortunate consequences. The deep breath, or conscious attention to breathing in any way, tends to turn into gasping or to result in some other kind of interference with the breathing involved in speaking. Scolding or punishment for "stuttering" usually brings on, fairly rapidly, aggravated hesitancy and tension. There are no such parental reactions as a rule, however, and in the average case the child shows only a gradual change in speech behavior. It is usually several months or even a year or two before he becomes a bit speech-shy, a little less talkative, a bit more hesitant, and a little strained, showing traces of effort in saying some words.

❡ ❡ ❡

In Study III we made a systematic effort to trace the development of the problem in each case. Even though there had been an average period of eighteen months, as nearly as we could determine, since the onset, nearly two thirds of the parents stated that at the time of our interview there was no tension in the child's speech as far as they could tell. Moreover, there had not been a great deal of change in the pattern of speech behavior that the parents regarded as stuttering. A few more children than at time of onset were prolonging the first sounds of words, which usually indicates some degree of strain, but most of them were still, the parents said, not doing this sort of thing. At onset "speech blocks" (we have discussed the problem of interpreting the meaning of this term) had been reported for three out of every hundred youngsters, and some eighteen months later, this number had increased to only six or seven out of every hundred. A few more were interjecting words or sounds like "well" or "uh uh," but there was not much difference between our clinical and control group children on this. The repetitions themselves were in some cases somewhat more tense, according to the parents, and the proportion of syllable repetitions, as compared with word and phrase repetitions, had increased a little during the year and a half between onset of the problem and our interview.

In addition to soliciting the parents' own observations of their children's speech, we attempted to obtain tape-recorded samples of the speech of the youngsters. Even though we worked in the homes of many of the children, particularly those in the control group, and in several different clinical centers, we managed to obtain clear and usable tape-recorded samples of the speech of most of the 150 pairs of children in Study III. By a pair I mean a control group child and a clinical group child, matched for age, sex, and social and economic level of family. We analyzed these speech samples and compared the two groups of children on several different measures of disfluency.

This analysis revealed certain differences between the two groups; there were also some interesting similarities; and there was much overlapping on most aspects of the comparison. For example, the two groups differed somewhat in the kinds of disfluency they showed most and least. For the control group most of the disfluencies were interjections ("uh uh uh") and revisions ("I was — I am going"); for the clinical group most of them were interjections and syllable and word repetitions. The two groups did about the same amount of interjecting of sounds like "uh uh," and, as has been noted, this was one of the most common types of disfluency for both groups. The two groups also showed about the same numbers of revisions, incomplete phrases, and broken words (the speaker starts to say a word, stops, pauses briefly, and then goes on to finish the word). They differed most in syllable and word repetitions and prolonged sounds and somewhat less in phrase repetitions, with the clinical group doing more of all these than the control group.

For the "stutterers" the median number of repetitions that involved either words or syllables was approximately six per hundred words, and for the "nonstutterers" the median number was between one and two per hundred words. The median numbers of all other kinds of disfluency were about seven for the clinical group and five for the control group per hundred words. No child in either group was perfectly fluent. The most disfluent child of those who were looked upon as normal speakers had eighteen breaks in fluency of one kind or another every hundred words, and half of them had over seven such breaks per hundred words. Half or more of those classified as stutterers had over thirteen disfluencies per hundred words.

The overlapping of the two groups was impressive. Taking the boys only (there were no statistically significant differences in speech fluency between the boys and girls in either group), and considering all types of disfluency combined, the most disfluent "nonstutterer" spoke less fluently than two thirds of the "stutterers." Twenty per cent of the "nonstutterers" were more disfluent than 30 per cent of the "stutterers." There was practically complete overlapping of the two groups for interjections, revisions, incomplete phrases, and broken words. There was more overlapping for phrase repetitions and prolonged sounds than for syllable and word repetitions. Even in syllable repetition, however, for which there was the largest average difference between the groups, the "nonstutterer" who did the most of this kind of repeating did more of it than 40 per cent of the "stutterers," and 20 per cent of all the "nonstutterers" did more repeating of syllables than did 20 per cent of all the "stutterers."

Thus, even though a child's parents regard him as a stutterer he may speak more fluently than many children who are looked upon by their parents as normal speakers. The problem called stuttering is not the same as the problem — when it is a problem — of disfluency. They are not completely different, or completely unrelated, but they are not one and the same.

◄ ◄ ◄

The findings we obtained by analyzing the tape-recordings are all the more striking because the speech samples we analyzed were not taken at the moment when, in each case, someone first regarded the child as a stutterer. The problem had been developing for a year and a half, on the average. For that period of time the children in the clinical group had been speaking in the face of parental concern and implied or expressed disapproval of the way they were talking, while those in the control group had been speaking presumably under normally favorable conditions.

Allowing for the possibility of some exceptions, certainly the majority of the children in the two groups were speaking with about equal fluency at the beginning of the eighteen-month period. The differences between the two groups that we observed at the end of that period indicate, therefore, the contrasting effects of the different conditions under which they had been talking during that time. Most of those whose attempts at speech had been regarded as stuttering and disapproved by their parents, however subtly and gently for the most part, had paid a price of some sort in increasing hesitancy, particularly in the form of more frequent repetition of the first parts of words and of whole words. Even so, many of them were still talking as fluently as were a considerable proportion of those who had not been classified as stutterers.

Our fluency analysis revealed one additional fact of major importance: in both groups the boys and girls were about equally fluent — or disfluent. Some girls speak more fluently than some boys, but substantial numbers of boys speak more fluently than a large proportion of girls. Traditionally it has been assumed that boys are not as fluent as girls, and that this accounts for the larger number of male stutterers. Now it turns out, according to our data, that there is apparently no greater disfluency in boys. This finding, moreover, agrees essentially with such other data as are available. All the relevant studies done to date have indicated that either there is no difference or else a relatively slight difference in speech fluency between very young members of the two sexes.

It is necessary, therefore, to explain on some other ground the fact that many more boys than girls are classified as stutterers. A good possibility is that we do not follow exactly the same policies and practices in raising boys and girls. The double standard may very well start in the cradle. If girls speak fully, or very nearly, as disfluently as boys do, and yet from about two and a half to four times more boys than girls are regarded as stutterers by their parents, this would seem to mean that parents do not judge the early speech of their little girls in quite the same way that they judge the early speech of their little boys. Here is something that requires further and very thorough investigation. Whatever it is that we are doing to little girls that results in fewer of them getting caught up in the problem of stuttering we should find out exactly what it is and start doing it to little boys too!

The problem called stuttering begins, then, when the child's speech is felt, usually by the mother, to be not as smooth or fluent as it ought to be. There seems as a rule to be a quality of puzzlement mixed with slight apprehension and dread about the mother's feeling. She uses the only name she knows for what she thinks must be the matter with her youngster's speech, and that word is "stuttering" — or, if she has grown up in England or certain other parts of the world, "stammering." Her first use of this word, however, may be rather loose and not very definite in meaning, at least as far as she is concerned. After all, as we have seen, in the most representative case the hesitations and repetitions she is calling "stuttering" are not very striking.

It is particularly to be noted that she had not noticed the disfluencies before, and so she thinks the youngster has just begun to do them. If he is doing the average number of about 50 every 1,000 words, they are likely to sound to her like a great — and sudden — lack of fluency. She may not be sure of herself at first in deciding that her child is stuttering, but her use of the word serves to crystallize her feelings and to focus her attention on the hesitations in the speech of her child. The more she attends to them and thinks about them as "stuttering," the more firm and deep becomes her conviction that the youngster is, indeed, a "stutterer" and that he has a grave problem.

All the while her feelings are becoming more and more clear to the child, and by a kind of process that we all commonly experience in one form or another but seldom try to put into words, he takes from his mother the feelings she has about his speech. In such a way he comes, slowly and by offs and ons, to doubt that he can get his words out "soon enough" and keep them coming smoothly one after another, and he learns to feel uneasy about this. Gradually, over a period of several months, in the usual case, this doubt and uneasiness affect him so that he loses some of his spontaneity in speaking and feels less like speaking at all and attempts it a little more hesitantly. In fact, after a while he no longer talks as much as he did before, especially to certain persons in certain places where his doubt and uneasiness are greatest.

Eventually he becomes hesitant enough in trying to say some things to some people that he holds back so much he has to force himself to go ahead, and this seems to be why he begins to speak with some degree of effort or strain. But to exert this effort he tenses up the muscles of his lips or tongue or throat and when he does this he talks even more hesitantly and less smoothly, and with some sense of difficulty, and as a result his doubt and uneasiness increase all the more. As a consequence he becomes more hesitant and holds back still more, and so he forces himself harder to go ahead, and in doing this he tenses his muscles increasingly, so that he speaks still less smoothly and with a greater sense of difficulty. On this distressing merry-go-round — or sad-go-round — his doubts and dreads are fed by his hesitations and tensions, which in turn are fed by his doubts and dreads.

While all this is happening to the child, his mother and father, and his sisters and his uncles and his aunts, and his playmates and his doctor and the ice cream man do not stand by idly and calmly. The less smoothly he speaks the more they worry, and the more they worry the more he senses their concern with the way he is speaking. The more he senses their concern the more uneasy he feels, and the more hesitantly and tensely he talks, the more they all worry — and this is an ever expanding spiral that carries everyone farther and farther from where they all want to be.

An unlucky seven out of every thousand children ride this sad-go-round into the adolescent years and beyond. They carry with them into adulthood the possibility of unhappiness and handicap that they would otherwise never know. The most sobering fact of all is that in all likelihood they — and their mothers and fathers and all their other companions in distress — need never have gone on this journey to nowhere that they had ever wanted to go. The best scientific information we have indicates, as I interpret it, that the problem we call stuttering is an avoidable accident.

We are left, however, with a most heartening prospect: through our continuing research and public education we may very well succeed in time in tearing down the old, old sad-go-round on which so many millions of the world's children and grownups are at this moment making their unrewarding way to ever more doubt and dread and tension. The glad promise of our findings to date is that the problem called stuttering can be prevented, and the learning of speech can be for every child a wonderful, wonderful ride on a merry-go-round of understanding and love and laughter.

CHAPTER *10*

How You Can Help Your Child

W HAT can be done for you — and by you — and other parents who must deal with the problem called stuttering?

Many of the things that can be done to reduce the problem after it has developed are the same things that can be done to prevent it in the first place. It is important, therefore, that these measures be made known not only to mothers and fathers who are already contending with stuttering, but also to the millions of young parents and parents-to-be who need never have the problem at all if only they are given essential information — and if they are enabled to make proper use of it.

Just how effective is the help that can be given to parents who are concerned that their children are stuttering? We can answer this question out of our general impressions as well as on the basis of research data. Our data as well as our impressions are to be weighed with a realistic sense of both their limitations and their usefulness in pointing the way to better understanding and more and more effective procedures.

It is often difficult to gauge the effects of clinical methods. There are many factors operating in any particular case, and we can control some of these but not others. Matters may become worse or better for reasons other than anything we may do. Good clinicians learn from experience simply to be as careful as possible in measuring and estimating the effects of their work, and to make good use of the most dependable information they can get to improve their methods as much as they can as they go along.

In the course of some of our studies of how the problem of stuttering begins we have given many of the parents a certain kind of counseling, and we have carried out investigations later to see what effects it had. In Chapter 3 we reviewed the findings of our follow-up study of the forty-six sets of parents who participated in the investigation we called Study I. After an average interval of about two and a half years following the first interview we attempted to find out in each case "how things were going." The results were very encouraging, especially when it is considered that while some of the parents were seen several times, many, for reasons that could not be controlled, received very little attention — and besides we were working without benefit of all that we have learned since the thirties.

In thirty-nine of the forty-six cases, or 85 per cent of the total group, either there had been improvement by the time we made our follow-up check or the problem no longer existed. Over half the children, twenty-five, or 54 per cent of the total group, were considered by everyone concerned to be speaking normally; in an additional eight cases there was some disagreement on whether speech was wholly normal or nearly so. Roughly seven out of ten, 72 per cent, were in these two classifications; six of the remaining thirteen children had improved.

Approximately twenty years later, in the fifties, we did another follow-up study of 118 cases from Study III. In forty-four of these it had been impossible for technical reasons to provide counseling for the parents, and in the other seventy-four cases the parents were given a very limited — practically minimal — amount of counseling. It was limited because it had to be worked in during the half-hour to an hour that was available in each case at the end of a tightly scheduled day of research interviewing and testing.

Even this small amount of counseling, plus the influence of the detailed interviewing itself, was evidently very worthwhile. You will recall that in Study III our research interview was carried out in the average case after the problem had persisted for about a year and a half. On the average, our follow-up investigation was made two years and a half after the research interview. At that time about nine out of ten of the children had improved or were no longer considered by their parents to have a speech problem. In only four cases had the problem become worse, ten were said to be "about the same," thirteen were reported to be somewhat better, forty-eight much better, and forty-three were judged by their mothers and fathers to be speaking normally.

These figures reflect the feelings of the parents. According to the two experienced speech pathologists who did the follow-up interviews, approximately 7 per cent of the children were still stutterers in a clinically significant sense, 15 per cent were "significantly disfluent" but not tense in speaking, and roughly three fourths were speaking with normal ease and fluency.

Moreover, a little counseling proved to be significantly better than none at all. We gathered data at three different clinical centers. Later we carried out follow-up interviews with forty-seven of the mothers who had been seen at Center A, twenty-seven who had been seen at Center B, and forty-four of those who had been interviewed originally at Center C. Those seen at Centers A and B had been given brief counseling, as has been indicated; no counseling had been provided at Center C. The proportion of children originally investigated in the three centers who were reported by their parents in the follow-up interviews to be speaking normally were, respectively, Center A 43 per cent, Center B 48 per cent (A and B combined, 45 per cent), and Center C 23 per cent. The difference between 45 and 23 per cent tests out to be a real difference, greater, that is, than could be accounted for by chance.

The clearest implication is that the counseling, brief though it was, made a difference. The fact that 23 per cent of those originally seen in Center C cleared up without benefit of parental counseling suggests rather strongly that the intensive interview done in Study III — answering the more than 800 questions took from three to five hours — proved to be in itself an enlightening and beneficial experience for the mothers and fathers who went through it. It made it possible for them to become more highly aware of "the facts in the case," and to take a full-length view of the development of the problem — and of their own part in it. These are steps that would be expected to lead nearly always to better understanding of the problem.

143

We compared the children who were said to be free of the problem at the time of the follow-up with those who were thought still to have a problem. Some of the similarities between the two groups were as interesting as the differences. For example, the Problem and No-Problem groups did not differ significantly with respect to proportions of boys and girls; the average length of time between the original research interview and the follow-up had been about the same for both groups; and the severity of the stuttering, as rated by both the parents and the clinical investigators, had been nearly the same on the average for both groups at the time of the original interview. After all, however, there were not many of the children in either group who were regarded as extremely severe stutterers in the first place, and it was the parents as much or more than the children who had the problem to overcome or not to overcome.

Among the most important differences between the Problem and No-Problem groups were these: those for whom the outcome had been very good — they no longer had a speech problem at the time of the follow-up — had been younger when they were first brought to the clinic, and the parents had not been concerned with the problem as long when they first sought clinical help. These findings indicate quite clearly that once the parents feel that the problem of stuttering exists, the sooner they obtain appropriate clinical services the better.

There were two other differences that seem deserving of a good deal of thought. One was that the mothers in the Problem group had indicated more concern over what they called their children's stuttering, and the other was that more of them had expressed concern over the impressions they made on other people. These two kinds of concern probably go together, and at least to some degree they apparently work against the chances of a good outcome for the problem.

The final difference we noted between the two groups seems particularly important. In the follow-up interview all the mothers were asked what advice they remembered receiving when they visited the clinic and how well they had carried it out. Although the two groups gave about the same sorts of accounts of the advice they had been given, significantly more of those who said they no longer had the problem — roughly two out of three as against two out of five — reported that they had carried out the recommendations "very thoroughly and consistently."

✎ ✎ ✎

It is only natural that you would be impatient to find out just what sort of counseling these two groups of parents were given. Before going into that, however, it is very important, I feel, that we look briefly at four additional sets of facts from which we have a great deal to learn about what might be helpful and not helpful to parents involved in this problem. Three of these we have already considered, and we have now to take a second look at them because of what they suggest concerning parental counseling.

First, fewer girls than boys get caught up in the problem called stuttering. As I have said, we should find out just what it is that we do to little girls that has this effect and start doing it to little boys too! Of course, so long as we take for granted that more boys than girls are classified as stutterers because boys talk less fluently, and that they talk less fluently because they are different from girls in some physical way that affects their speech in this specific sense — well, it doesn't occur to us to wonder whether there could be some other explanation. As we have seen, however, analysis of our tape-recorded speech samples did not show that boys speak significantly less fluently than girls. This finding makes it very hard for us to hang on to the idea that more boys than girls are classified by their parents as stutterers because of some physical characteristic of boys that makes them repeat and hesitate much more in speaking. The basic fact from which we have something very fundamental to learn is that, on the contrary, two to four times more boys than girls are regarded by their parents as stutterers *in spite of the fact* that there is little or no difference between them generally in fluency of speech. This is, indeed, a thought-provoking fact. It suggests that we do not treat girl and boy toddlers alike.

Second, there is a large group of children who are seldom classified as stutterers — boys and girls who are very young, below roughly the age of two and one-half years. Now, one of the most important things about these very young children is that they do not speak as fluently on the average as those who are one to two years older, and in spite of this they are much less often regarded as stutterers than are the older and more fluent youngsters. The old, and still common, idea that the less fluent a child is the more likely he is to be tagged as a stutterer does not account for this situation. Again it is to be said that we should find out what it is that we do to our two-year-olds that explains why we do not tend to create the problem of stuttering for them, and start doing it to our three- and four-year-olds too.

Third, you will recall the "stuttering Simpsons" in Chapter 5. In the fourth and fifth generations, you will remember, one out of every three children was a stutterer. This was during the time when the Simpsons took for granted that stuttering was hereditary in their family, and they acted on this belief in observing and evaluating the disfluencies in the speech of their small children. Then, some twenty years ago, we made a study of the family and in doing so we brought to them new information that they had not known about before, and new ways of looking at their youngsters' speech hesitations, which resulted in their developing new ways of feeling about them and judging them. And now, among forty-four children in the sixth generation there is not even one who has become involved in the problem called stuttering. It is to be said, again, that whatever the parents of the sixth generation of Simpsons have been doing to their youngsters, we should find out what it is and do it to all our other children too.

A fourth point, which we have not considered before, concerns the Ute, the Bannock, and the Shoshone Indians, and possibly other societies as well, who do not have the problem we call stuttering, or indeed a word for it. (See Chapter 17, "The Indians Have No Word For It," of my *People in Quandaries*.) We first came upon this rather startling and highly significant fact about twenty years ago, when I suggested to one of my graduate students, Miss Harriett Hayes, that she make a study of stutterers among the Bannock and Shoshone children in the school in which she was going to be teaching in Idaho. She left Iowa one September with detailed plans for such a study — and returned from Idaho the following June with the seemingly

146

strange information that not only had she been unable to find any stutterers of whom to make a study among the Bannock and Shoshone, but she had also made extensive inquiries and had not succeeded in locating anyone who had ever known of a stutterer among the members of these two tribes. What seemed most intriguing was the report by Miss Hayes that these Indians had no word for "stuttering."

Later another of my students, Dr. John Snidecor, extended the investigation in Idaho and thoroughly confirmed the finding that the Bannock and Shoshone had neither the problem nor the word "stuttering." He also reported that they seemed to take practically no notice of disfluency in their children's speech, and that in general their child-rearing practices were more lax and less demanding than our own.

Meantime other investigators became interested in the question of cultural variations in the prevalence of stuttering. Dr. John Morgenstern completed a study at the University of Edinburgh in 1953 in which he determined that a number of more or less "undeveloped" societies in various parts of the world do not know stuttering. With absence of the problem there goes consistently an absence also of a word for the problem. It is not that the children in these societies speak perfectly fluently and so have no hesitations to be classified as stuttering; it seems, rather, that the absence of a word like "stuttering" indicates that the parents attach no importance to their children's disfluencies and so feel no need to make the judgment that some of them, or any of them, in the speech of some children are "too many or too much." It also seems that the presence of such a word in a language makes more likely that some parents will use it to point up a distinction between the speech of some children and that of others.

The most intensive investigation of this type to date was published in 1961 by Dr. Joseph Stewart. The anthropologist Dr. David Stout shared with me the supervision of this research. Dr. Stewart carried out a systematic field study among the Ute Indians in Utah and certain other groups of North American Indians in Vancouver. The Indians of Vancouver were selected for investigation because they reportedly did have the stuttering problem, and the Ute were chosen

147

for comparison because they reportedly did not. Dr. Stewart found that the problem was indeed unknown among the Ute, that they had no word for it, and that their child-rearing practices were such that no issue was made of the children's disfluencies in speaking.

He found that among the Indians of Vancouver there had been a much greater prevalence of stuttering two generations ago than there is today, and that it had been associated with intense social and economic competition among the families. This competition included especially a great deal of ceremonial speaking on occasions of social importance. The young children took part in this ceremonial speaking, under pain of deep humiliation for themselves and their families if they made mistakes. These customs began to change many years ago as the Indians' way of life was altered by economic changes, and the ceremonial speaking and related competitive social practices have now all but died out. As they have gone, so too the problem of stuttering has very greatly decreased, and Dr. Stewart found that most of the Indians he interviewed in Vancouver were not familiar with the old word for "stuttering" and had not used it for many years.

◀ ◀ ◀

What, then, are the great lessons we have to learn from such cultures as those of the Ute, Bannock, and Shoshone, from such families as the Simpsons, and from a greater awareness of what we ourselves do to our own very young boys and girls, and to our little girls when they are slightly older than very young, that prevents or greatly limits the problem called stuttering? And what have we learned that can be passed on to you from the very encouraging experience we have had in the past twenty-five years or so in counseling parents faced with the problem called stuttering?

By all odds the greatest lesson we all have to learn is this: When we come somehow to doubt that a child has the ability "to get his words out soon enough" or to talk as smoothly as, for some reason, we think he should, he catches our doubt and becomes himself infected by it. When we allow our doubt to worry us, the child is infected by our worry. Doubt and uneasiness are as contagious as mumps and measles. They are carried by words and glances as swiftly as bacteria are carried by the wind. But their effects can be far more lasting and in their own peculiar ways ever so much more disabling.

Just as we have learned to protect our children against most bacteria, so we can learn to give them immunity against unjustified doubt about themselves and the unwholesome feelings and tensions that it breeds. To do this we need in the main two things: enough dependable information and a proper sense of values.

From the inspiring story of the "no longer stuttering Simpsons" we can learn, if we will, that if we are to make use of new knowledge and gain new perspectives we must give up, as they did gladly, old beliefs and feelings. If we are to equal the wisdom of the Ute and eliminate the problem of stuttering from our own culture, we must cease to take for granted that stuttering — not a certain amount of disfluency, but *stuttering* — is unavoidably the fate by birth, or by the accident of illness or injury or emotional distress, of a certain proportion of our children, generation in and generation out, until the Earth shall cool. The belief that any specific child is doomed by some sort of inborn or acquired predisposition to "be a stutterer" is not good for the child unless it is an honest facing up to undeniable evidence. As a routine assumption it is a doctrine of despair. After due examination we may conclude that, because of brain damage perhaps, or some more temporary cause, a particular child may not be expected to speak with ordinary or average fluency; this is not to say, however, that he must become involved in the unfavorable reactions of other persons and the resultant discontents and tensions that make up the problem we call stuttering. It is only to say that for a time, or indefinitely, he may not speak as fluently as most other children, or older persons, do. The degree of fluency, or of disfluency, with which a child speaks is one thing; whether or not we classify the way he speaks as "abnormal," or as "stuttering," and regard him as a "stutterer," is something else again, something very different indeed.

◀   ◀   ◀

The counseling we gave the parents in Study I and Study III was about like that we gave the parents of the fourth generation of Simpsons, whose twenty-four children in the fifth generation, the eight who stuttered together with the rest, have grown up to bring into the world forty-four children of their own who are happily free of the distress and handicap of being classified as stutterers. The counseling may be summarized by saying that we began in each case by leading the parents through an interview that made it possible for them to review in an orderly and objective fashion, and in detail, the course of the problem since they had first persuaded themselves of its presence. It is the common experience of specialists who work with problems of feeling and thinking and behavior — as distinguished from physical diseases and injuries — that the basic act of facing up to a problem, retracing the pattern of events and taking a good long look at the facts, is at least half the battle. My own experience has convinced me that this is undoubtedly true in working with parents who are concerned with what they regard as stuttering.

What the parents in our studies told us — and in doing so told themselves — has been summed up in the preceding chapters of this book. A steady viewing of the facts in these cases is reassuring. The problem we call stuttering is definitely magnified by the worrying we — you and other parents and everyone concerned — do about it. In part this is true because we go off away from the facts to do our worrying. It is not that we worry very much, if at all, about what the child actually has done in any specific situation in response to the particular conditions that were there for him to respond to at the time. We worry, instead, about our particular memory of what he may have done and our special interpretation of it, as well as our beliefs concerning it. We worry because we tend to forget or to disregard the time, the place, and the circumstances. And we become concerned because we forget, or have never known, just how much the things our child sometimes does are like the things other children sometimes do under similar conditions. We worry because we tend to focus on one thing — the repeating or hesitating our child does — to the exclusion of nearly everything else. It is the "everything else" that makes his repeating and hesitating understandable and even unremarkable.

What happens, then, when we review the facts — if we take enough

150

time for it, something like two to five or six hours, at least, plus the many days or weeks or months it takes us to think them through — is that we gain, or recapture, a needed perspective. We see things in their proper relationships to other things. The foreground detail that we have pulled out of the picture and concentrated on we now put back where it belongs, against the background of the total picture, and we see it in a way that enlightens us more and frightens us less. The interviewing we did in order to get the history of the problem in each case was, therefore, a very important part of the counseling process. I think that goes far to account for the fact that even those parents who had no counseling in addition to this reported, nevertheless, in most of the follow-up studies that things had improved or that, in nearly a fourth of the cases, there was no longer any problem at all.

In addition to helping the parents review the facts objectively and take in the parts of the total picture that they had been disregarding, we tried to do essentially three things. First, we gave the parents as much information as we could under the circumstances about normal speech development in young children. We told them about the conditions that affect it badly and favorably. We talked with them about the problem of stuttering and the facts of its onset and development in the general run of cases. Second, we helped them to point up the facts that seemed to be most important in their own case. Third, we tried to work out with them some practical suggestions for making good use, in their day-to-day thinking and practices in their own homes, of the things they had learned from the clinical experience they had just been through.

This book has been intended, up to this point, to help you achieve, among other things, the first of these objectives, so far as you could do this by means of a book. We have accomplished the second part of the counseling process also, as well as we could through the medium of the printed page, if, as you have read this book, you have thought about your own child and yourself and your own problem, making the book speak to you specifically about you and your child in every way you could. What remains to be done, then, is to help you put into practice what you have learned so far by spelling out for you the practical suggestions you might apply in your own home day in and day out, and from minute to minute, in everything you think and feel and do that concerns your child's speech.

◆ ◆ ◆

First: *Make no issue of your child's repetitions and hesitations in speaking.*

The basic fact to keep firmly in mind is that repetitions and other kinds of hesitation are part and parcel of normal speech. The sweetest sound your child has ever made, the cry of birth, is one that he repeated over and over again. You may not have noticed that it was repeated — because you were distracted by the happiness it gave you. If your child is like most other children he repeated about half of all the vocal sounds he made during his first year of life. When he began to form his sounds into words he did not stop repeating them, and he also repeated the words sometimes. When he began to put the words together to make phrases and sentences, he repeated some of those as well. This was no simple trick, making words out of sounds and sentences out of words, and your youngster did a certain amount of fumbling in learning how to do it. Like the rest of us, he will continue to fumble with words more or less all his life.

Then, too, it was by learning to say words *to other people* that your child pecked his way out of the shell of his original self-absorption into the confusingly bright light of what we call the social world of give and take. As he was learning to speak, that is, he was also learning to respond with speech to more and more other people and to figure out what to make of their reactions to the things he said to them. He did not do this, of course, without some feelings of uncertainty, even some tensions now and then, and he sometimes stood for a while first on one verbal foot and then on the other before going ahead. And again, like the rest of us, he will go on doing this to some extent in his own way and for his own reasons so long as he relates himself to other human beings by talking with them.

If no issue is made by you or the child's other listeners of the repetitions and hesitations in his speech, the child himself is not at all likely to make an issue of them. This means that they will simply be accepted or passed over by you and others and taken in stride, or not be noticed at all, by the youngster — and nothing will come of them. I know of no reason why the particular problem that is called stuttering need ever arise for you or your child if (a) the child's listeners — and you, his parents, are by all odds his most important listeners — never begin to think he ought to speak more fluently than he does, (b) you never begin to consider his repetitions and hesitations "undesirable" or "abnormal," and (c) you never begin to classify them as "stuttering" and react to them accordingly with uneasiness and worry, which sooner or later in one way or another you would unavoidably make known to the youngster. It is the distinctive mark of the problem we call stuttering that it does involve such feelings and the reactions to which they give rise — first in the listener and later in the speaking child who learns, or catches, them from the listener. In the absence of these distinctive feelings and their unique effects, speech may be more or less disfluent, and even tense, but the pattern of feeling and behavior, and of interactions between listener and speaker, that distinguishes stuttering — in a significant clinical sense of the word — can hardly be said to exist.

What can be true meanwhile — and this is a very different matter, indeed — is that at times your child may repeat and hesitate decidedly more than most other children do, and some of the ways in which he does these things may be different from the ways in which most other children do them. If this is the case, it is still to be stressed that no issue should be made of your child's repetitions and hesitations, as such. The issue, if there is to be one, should be made of the conditions that are responsible for the youngster's unusually disfluent speech. By his extraordinary hesitations — if they are, in fact, extraordinary — your child is directing your attention, if you will but look, from his mouth, from his speech itself, to something or other he is reacting to that should be found and changed or eliminated. But, first of all and above all, be very sure that what you take to be unusual disfluency really is unusual.

What is an unusual amount of disfluency? One answer to this question is to be found in the analysis we made of tape-recorded speech samples from the children in Study III. You will recall that the youngsters ranged in age from a little under three to about eight years. We obtained samples of their speech by having them talk about a set of pictures. We identified and counted eight different kinds of disfluency in their speech.

The least fluent boy in the control group was disfluent in one way or another 183 times every 1,000 words on the average. This might seem extreme, especially in view of the fact that even two thirds of the so-called stuttering children spoke more fluently than this boy did — and yet he was not regarded by anyone as a stutterer. The least fluent girl who was looked upon as a normal speaker was disfluent in some way 287 times every 1,000 words, more frequently than all but about 10 per cent of the girls who were regarded by their parents as stutterers.

A rough gauge in a statistical sense might be provided by saying that the least fluent one fourth of the children whose speech was taken to be normal spoke with about 100 disfluencies per 1,000 words, or one for every ten words.* It is to be emphasized, of course, that although this may seem to some listeners to be a great deal of disfluency, none of these children was thought of by anyone as a stutterer. At the same time, curiously enough, some three out of ten of the youngsters who were looked upon as stutterers were speaking more fluently than they were.

It is most difficult, therefore, to say just what is "an extreme amount" of disfluency in any objective sense — at least in any meaningful relationship to the question of whether there are some amounts of disfluency that "should be called stuttering." But, then, this question itself would hardly seem to be very meaningful. What it comes down to is that among children who are regarded as normal speakers, some are more disfluent than others, and still others are a great deal

---

* In the analysis described here we did not count any word more than once, in computing the total number of words in a sample, so that a repeated word, such such such as that, was counted not as three words but only as one. In other studies (see Chapter 4 of *Stuttering in Children and Adults*) we did count each repetition of a word as a word, counting such such such, for example, as three words. This difference in method of computing the total number of words accounts largely for the variations in the findings, in terms of the number of disfluencies per 100 words, or 1,000 words, from one study to another.

more disfluent than some; but they are all accepted as normal speakers by their parents as well as by everybody else.

What *kinds* of disfluency are unusual? Again, we can look to our children's tape-recorded speech samples for a kind of answer. In the speech of the children looked upon as normal speakers somewhat over 90 per cent of the disfluencies were interjections ("uh well uh"), repetitions of sounds, words, or phrases, and revisions ("I am — I was going"). At the same time, however, these types accounted for nearly the same proportion of the disfluencies in the speech of the so-called stutterers. After all, there are just so many things a child — or a grownup — can do to interrupt his speech.

By going into finer detail we can tease out some differences between the two groups. It will be recalled that the children called stutterers did relatively more repeating of syllables than of words, and those called normal speakers did relatively more repeating of words than of syllables. There was not much difference so far as phrase repetitions were concerned. You will also remember that there were two other fairly clear differences: the children regarded as stutterers did more prolonging of sounds, as in dragging out the first sound of a word l . . . ike that, but this was among the less frequent types of disfluency for both groups; and the control group children did relatively more interjecting of sounds and words ("uh well uh") than did those in the clinical group, although for both groups this was one of the most common types of disfluency.

It is to be borne in mind, of course, that our speech samples were recorded about eighteen months, on the average, after the problem of stuttering was said to have arisen. So far as we could determine, the two groups of children must have been speaking very much alike at the start of that period. Apparently, then, the differences between the two groups were due chiefly, if not entirely, to the fact that the clinical group children had been speaking for eighteen months under conditions of parental disapproval of their speech, while the control group children had been speaking under the more favorable conditions of having their speech generally accepted. The experience of speaking for that period of time in the face of more or less negative listener reactions had evidently influenced the clinical group young-

155

sters to speak, on the average, somewhat more hesitantly. They not only repeated or hesitated more often, but also apparently with slightly more tension in some cases. As a child comes to be more doubtful and concerned about his ability to say his words "soon enough or smoothly enough," it seems likely that he will shift, as the clinical group children did to some extent, from the more relaxed hesitation forms of word and phrase repetition, and the interjection of "uh uh" and the like, to the more tense or less leisurely hesitations involved in dragging out or repeating the first sounds of words. Even so, it is to be recalled that, according to our speech analysis as well as the parents' interviews, there were also hesitations and repetitions that were more or less tense in the speech of some of the children regarded as normal speakers. There is, then, no sharp line between hesitations that are and those that are not "unusual" in form.

In view of these facts, it would hardly be wise to define "unusual amount and kind of disfluency" with unrealistic precision. I doubt that most parents could do much better than to follow some such rough rule as this: If a child is hesitating and repeating in ways that seem tense or strained, or if he seems to be speaking much more disfluently than most other children of his age, attention should be given to the possible reasons, including especially those outside the child. It should not be taken for granted that anything is wrong with the child's body, or personality, or with his speech, as such. Rather, the best working assumption is that he is speaking in a way normally to be expected under the circumstances — and that it is the circumstances that are to be investigated and changed in any ways that seem desirable or necessary.

If you follow this practical rule, you begin by assuming — on the firm basis of research findings and clinical experience to date — that your child is physically able to speak with normal fluency under conditions that make normal speech possible or likely. You will assume, therefore, that if he does not seem to be speaking with normal (not perfect) fluency at all times the conditions under which he is speaking are not wholly favorable.

Dr. Dean Williams has shown that when parents are advised to keep an ear out for the *normal* hesitations and repetitions in their children's speech, they tend clearly to classify more and more of the disfluencies as normal and correspondingly fewer of them as "stuttering." The net effect is that the way the children are speaking seems better and better to the parents. As their concern is reduced accordingly, they become easier for their youngsters to talk to — and so the children not only seem to speak, but actually do speak, with less hesitancy and more freely and confidently. This re-focusing of the parents' attention often proves, therefore, to be a particularly effective aid in breaking up the vicious circle of hesitancy, concern, more hesitancy, more concern, etc. You would doubtless be well advised, therefore, to employ this suggestion and listen particularly for the hesitations and repetitions in your child's speech that you would regard as normal.

If you do this, and if you follow the other recommendations in this chapter, it is to be expected that you will less and less frequently raise the question of whether your youngster is "stuttering" or is a "stutterer." No good can possibly come, and harm can surely result, from raising this question. You will ask, rather, whether your youngster might talk more fluently and freely if certain changes were made in the circumstances under which he is speaking. But you will be very liberal in the amount of disfluency you call reasonable. You will take a lesson from the Ute and Bannock and Shoshone and lean far toward the side of making no issue at all of your child's repetitions and hesitations. You will keep in mind the "no longer stuttering Simpsons" and feel, as they happily learned to feel, that it is far better that your child speak with pleasure than with fluency.

If, however, you have applied as best you can all the lessons you have learned from these pages so far, and you feel that there is something to be gained by seeing what you can do to improve the conditions under which your child is speaking, then you will want to know what to look for and what to change in order to improve them.

⤳   ⤳   ⤳

Second: *Eliminate or modify any conditions that tend to make your child speak with unusual amounts or kinds of repetition and hesitation.*

In general, children speak less fluently and more tensely under the following conditions:

a. When they are very excited.

b. When they are speaking in a great hurry.

c. When they are competing with others who are speaking and find it hard to get a word in edgewise — and so when they do they tend to "hold the floor" by repeating what they have said until they can think of what to say next.

d. When they are speaking to listeners who are not paying much attention to them, such as a father who is engrossed in the stock market quotations or a mother figuring out a complicated dress pattern.

e. When they are "talking over their heads," groping for words when they don't quite know what they are talking about, or are not familiar with the words they need in order to say what they do know.

f. When they are speaking under excessive restrictions, as under the influence of a father who "wants some peace and quiet" so he can rest, or a mother whose vocabulary seems to consist mostly of "No!" "Stop that!" "Don't do that!" and "I've just cleaned the living room so don't go in there with your bubble gum and modeling clay!"

g. When they are trying to speak under the stress of fright, shame, dread, embarrassment, and other strong emotions, especially those that are depressing or demoralizing. Such experiences are for the most part unavoidable, within limits, even in the best-run families, and so the point is not to try to eliminate them completely but to appreciate the effects they tend to have on the child's speech when they occur. In anger, incidentally, children, like adults, sometimes speak with great fluency, at other times with equally great disruption, amounting even to speechlessness.

h. When — and this is the most important condition of all — they are speaking to parents, or other important listeners such as grandparents or teachers, who seem "hard to please" because they have high standards and are rather perfectionistic, especially about speech fluency itself. Children tend to be particularly hesitant in speaking to listeners by whom they are looked upon as "stutterers." They may not know in any clear or technical sense that what they are doing is being "classified as stuttering," but they easily sense that something is wrong. Children are as sharp as puppies at detecting our real feelings about them. It is as difficult for them as it would be for any of us to talk freely, spontaneously, and smoothly to someone who seems to be feeling that there is something the matter with *the way* they are talking. If, whenever you were to hesitate or to repeat word, someone very important to you were to give some sign o questioning or concern, a glance, a sudden looking away, an unusua. movement, you know, of course, the slowly growing uneasiness you would feel, and the sense of uncertainty and hesitation and conflict with which you would come to speak. The feelings and reactions of a child under such conditions are not at all difficult for us to understand, once we put ourselves in his place as best we can, and let ourselves be sensitive to the reasons for his doubt and hesitation and tension.

Although all these conditions, except the last one, are more or less ordinary, one or another of them can become extreme in almost any home now and then. For example, there are fathers who very seldom seem to pay any attention to what their children are trying to tell them. I have actually encouraged a few fathers of this sort to get down on the floor with their small children and not only listen to them but play and romp with them as well, and I am sure that both the fathers and the youngsters were much the better for it.

I have seen a few parents, mostly fathers, who seem to think it is jolly fun and good for the kiddies to be wrestled and teased until they are too excited and breathless to say four words in a row and finally collapse from utter exhaustion. Older children are sometimes allowed to keep younger ones in a state of excitement beyond reasonable limits. Hearty playfulness is one thing, but screaming abandon is something entirely different for which there is practically nothing good to be said.

One mother reported that her little three-year-old boy seemed to speak with much more than usual repeating whenever she went to his nursery school to bring him home for lunch. What happened at those times, we found, was that he wanted to show her things he had made, but she had almost always left something on the stove or for some other reason felt under pressure to hurry back home again. He would practically drag her by the hand about the little school to show her and tell her about the coloring he had done and the things he had built with blocks, and all the while she was holding back and telling him to hurry up, that the beans would burn, that they had to go quickly, and he was hurriedly groping for words and filling in with uh's and er's and um's and doing far more repeating and hesitating than most other children do, or than he himself did as a rule. I suggested that she simply leave for the nursery school ten minutes sooner, turning off the gas before she left, and give the little fellow enough time to show her and tell her about the things he wanted to share with her. As was to be expected, of course, the resulting change in his speech was remarkable.

There are times when a child just doesn't have the words he needs. I have a vivid memory of one three-year-old boy telling at the dinner table one evening about something he had seen in a neighbor's basement that afternoon. With all the gestures he would have used in a game of charades he attempted with earnestness and persistence to explain that "it was uh well uh um ah so high and uh er uh uh so long and it was uh uh" — well, it turned out to have been a hobby horse, and he had never seen such a thing before and he had no idea what it was called. As soon as he was given the name "hobby horse" he settled down immediately to his usual verbal pace.

If you are like most other parents it would probably pay you to try, just on general principles, to reduce the No's and Don't's with which you influence your child. Every Do you use removes the necessity for at least two or three Don't's. Besides, a certain proportion of the No's and Don't's do not have to be replaced with Do's because they are unnecessary and can simply be eliminated. They are spoken almost by reflex out of deeply grooved habit. A little more accent on the positive is usually possible and always beneficial not only to your child but fully as much to yourself as well.

One case that I have described before (in *Speech Handicapped School Children*) illustrates so many of the conditions that can be reduced or eliminated in the interests of more fluent and generally better speech that I should like to tell about it again. This was the story of little four-year-old Chuck, who was definitely doing an excessive amount of repeating and showing some degree of tension at times. Investigation turned up a long list of conditions under which he was speaking with a good deal of hesitation and repetition, because Chuck's mother, Mrs. Carter, was carrying on a "running fight" with him. She was fussing with him at the table about the foods he wouldn't eat, and about the way he ate the foods he would eat; in trying to get him to nap she wrestled with him every afternoon, and bedtime was another battle scene; whenever he ran to the neighbors she called him back, or went and brought him back, usually against lively resistance; and in addition he liked to "pound" the piano, but his father, who was a musician and "couldn't stand it," habitually insisted that he stop. There were other details.

A program was worked out for changing all this. The mother was to ignore Chuck's eating habits, at least temporarily. The afternoon naps were to be discontinued. Stories were to be read at bedtime. In addition, Chuck was to be allowed much more freedom in going about the neighborhood. Mrs. Carter was to talk to the neighbors and explain that if Chuck caused them any inconvenience she would appreciate their calling her; otherwise, he was to be free to come and go and play with the other children. A particularly happy touch was that instead of resenting Chuck's "pounding" the father was to teach him how to play the piano — an idea which had never occurred to him and which he thought was splendid.

In order to get the whole plan properly launched Mrs. Carter was to spend a day at the city park with Chuck. She was to "talk it up" for at least three days, planning with Chuck just how they would go, what they would do when they got there, what things they would take along, what they would carry in the lunch basket, whether to include orangeade or chocolate milk, and so on and on. Then when the Big Day came they were really to go and spend the whole day, just the two of them. Chuck was to be allowed to play as he liked to his heart's content. The mother was to watch over his physical safety, of course, but gently and with no scolding whatever. Then, next morning, as soon as he came down to breakfast, Mrs. Carter was to start a lively conversation about all the fun they had had the day before, and she was to keep referring to it at every reasonable opportu-

161

nity. And more good times were to be planned and carried through and talked about at great length.

This was done, and it made a tremendous difference. For a year or so Chuck had been speaking with considerable disfluency; the circumstances were such that almost any child would have. On top of everything else, the Carters had come several months before to think of what Chuck was doing as stuttering, and this had greatly complicated an already unfavorable situation and made it worse. As a consequence Chuck had developed some pretty tense and hesitant speech reactions by the time we were called in. Within two months after we got "the plan" underway, however, Mrs. Carter reported that the speech problem had cleared up, that Chuck's behavior — as well as her own — had improved generally, and that "you wouldn't recognize this home as the same place any more."

The basic consideration is that if he is hesitating and repeating beyond reasonable limits, your child, any child, is responding to a situation. It is the situation that needs to be examined and "diagnosed." It is the situation that needs to be "treated." In fact, your child's speech is likely to smooth out to some degree almost as soon as you take your attention off his disfluency and start observing as best you can the specific things — including your own attitudes and practices — to which he is responding hesitantly and tensely. And you will discover that with few exceptions you are able to make the changes that you find should be made.

As has been stressed repeatedly, the most important condition of all, of course, under which a child tends to speak with exaggerated hesitancy and strain is that one which his parents accidentally and with the best of intentions create for him when they classify the ordinary — or extraordinary — repeating and hesitating he does as "abnormal" and as "stuttering," and so come to look upon him as a "stutterer." When they make these judgments of him and of what he does when he speaks they unwittingly, and against their deepest desires, affect in unfortunate ways the relationship they have with him. They become innocently the sort of listeners with whom he feels a little less sure of himself, and so he gradually comes to speak a little more hesitantly to them. As others accept their judgment of him and his speech, and are influenced by their concern, they react accordingly, and so the child comes to speak a bit more hesitantly to them too. When he has become hesitant enough he experiences the conflict that comes from having to force himself to speak because he feels so much like holding back, and with this comes the tension and all that goes with it to make up a sort of speech behavior that no one would wish for any child.

Conditions that have been or that are being created in this way are the main ones to be looked for — and, most especially, to be completely avoided — in any case. If they have not been avoided they should be recognized, understood as clearly as thorough investigation and self-searching will permit, and eliminated as fully as possible. In fact, if these particular conditions can be avoided or eliminated, it is extremely unlikely, if not wholly impossible, that stuttering, as this word has meaning in a significant clinical sense, will ever be a problem for you and your child, although he may at times speak very haltingly, even tensely, for other reasons.

Some of the ways in which you can work toward these objectives have been described and implied in the past few pages. There are other ways, too, and we shall now consider them.

◀ ◀ ◀

Third: *Do everything you can to make speaking rewarding and fun for your child.*

If your responses to the talking your child does to you are satisfying to him, he will want to talk to you all the more, and he will in fact do more talking to you because he will enjoy it. And he is likely to feel toward other people and to react to them pretty much as he feels toward you and reacts to you. If in the time he spends with you he learns to enjoy talking, the chances are very good indeed that he will find pleasure in talking to just about everybody else as well.

Now, if your child enjoys talking because he finds that speaking is satisfying and makes things go better and adds pleasure and adventure and accomplishment to his minutes and hours and days, he will have no compelling reason to doubt that he can or should speak. Without such doubt and the uneasiness that goes with it, he will

163

simply speak as smoothly *or as hesitantly* as is natural and normal in view of his state of calmness or excitement, vigor or fatigue, interest or boredom, friendliness or antagonism, and in view of the circumstances he is in at the moment — whether he is being interrupted or heckled or "talked down" by others, or is being ignored or listened to with interest and appreciation; whether he has to search and fumble for words or has adequate vocabulary for expressing what he has to tell, is in new and bewildering surroundings or old and familiar territory; whether he is being influenced by one or another of ever so many things that make a difference in the fluency of his speech, just as they affect the fluency of your speech or that of anyone else.

¶ ¶ ¶

Fourth: *Do everything you can to be a good listener for your child.*

The one thing you can do that will go farthest, in my judgment, to ensure that your child will grow up to be the clear-eyed, considerate, constructive person you want him to become is to teach him to be a good listener. The surest way to do that is to set him an example by being a good listener yourself. In the bargain, you will be doing one of the most important things you could ever do to make the speaking he does to you rewarding and enjoyable. And — this is indeed a surprise package filled with riches — you will be improving your own relationship, not only with your youngster, which would be wonderful enough, but also with the butcher and the baker and the candlestick maker and your seat neighbors on the subway and the bus, with advantages beyond anything you could possibly predict.

In saying this I realize that you may feel I am giving you more answer than you asked for, that I am going far beyond telling you how to keep your child from being caught up in, or how to remove him from, the problem called stuttering. The wonderful truth is, however, that one thing leads to another. You just cannot do the right things for your child without hitting a jackpot of blessings. Your cup runneth over unavoidably if your child enjoys talking with you because you like to listen to him.

If you are a good listener you hear your child out. Granted, it takes a little time — sometimes — but the things you learn about your youngster and his strange and wonderful world, and the pleasures you have doing it, are beyond any price you could ever pay by spending the time it takes.

If you are a good listener you draw your child out. You do this by hanging on his words, by looking interested because you really are interested, and by asking questions like "Well, how *big* was it and was it green *all over*?" and "Yes, but *how* could you tell it was alive?" and "Oh, I see, but *where did* the ants get in?"

If you are a good listener you take what your child says without batting an eye — when most people would. You wonder sometimes why he would ever say the things he does, but the point is you do wonder about it. You don't just shush him. Maybe he's imagining things, some pretty fantastic things, but imagination is a wonderful, wonderful gift that flourishes with use — and just a little careful questioning now and then. Or maybe he's trying to tell you that he feels put upon, irritated, and outraged, and if you listen closely enough you might find out what his reasons are, and then you can do something about them if they seem important, or something about his way of looking at them if they don't.

If you are a good listener for your child it is because you want to share his wonderment and joys and hurts, to feel again as fully as you can what it's like to be so small — and to grow up so fast that there is hardly ever time enough just to be as young as you are. And so, if you are a good listener, your child will not only find it easy and good to talk with you, but he will enjoy listening to you too, and when he has grown up surely he will remember you as the best mother or father in all the world. And no one who understands will ever question the truth of this — because the truth of it can only be his to know.

❧ ❧ ❧

Fifth: *Do everything you can to make speech a personal sharing for you and your child.*

Speaking will be more rewarding and enjoyable for your child as it comes to be for him more and more a way of sharing himself with you and others — and again he will learn more by example than in any other way. If in speaking to your youngster you share yourself with him he will learn to share himself when he talks with you. And the talking he learns to do with you he will tend to carry over into the speaking he does with others too. He will make friends wherever he goes, because he will be understanding and understandable, if he can share with other people, and help them to share with him, the regrets and joys and dreads and hopes in which they find themselves to be reassuringly alike and excitingly different.

To be a personal sharing speech must be sincere. You cannot share yourself with a small child by talking down to him. You do it best by saying what you mean as clearly as you can, and by trying to explain why you can't be more clear. This means you do it best not only when you speak with kindness and delight, but also — and this should not be surprising — when you speak in anger or discouragement, out of annoyance or grief, and, sometimes at least, in tones of criticism and urgent instruction. Some parents seem to have forgotten — perhaps there are some who have never realized — that one way to reject a child is never to say a hasty word to him, never to scold or criticize him, never to raise a hand or a voice in the age-old ways that tell a child beyond question that you care about him and what is to become of him.

One of my former students is a teacher in a school for crippled children in one of our larger cities, and she told me one time a story that I can never forget. Perhaps if I share it with you it will haunt your memory, too, and increase by so much the immortality of a little girl who surely could not have known how wise she was in her delight. Mary Lou was nine, and she could barely get about slowly with braces because of the aftereffects of polio. One morning she came to school with her brown eyes bright and her face glowing with happiness. She had nothing but smiles for everyone. The other children could do no wrong and all was right in the little world of Mary Lou. When the teacher could contain her curiosity no longer she asked her why in the world she felt so good, and Mary Lou answered in words that all but sang: "Something wonderful happened to me last night! I got my first spanking!"

What matters above all is that we care, and if we care enough our children know we do — because we make our meaning very clear.

We do forget sometimes that mere words are not always easy to understand. There are times when a child can understand them only if we speak them with italics, as it were, and underlining, and with exclamation points. And when words, spoken as effectively as we can utter them, are beyond a child's comprehension, love finds some other way to reach his understanding.

It is important that we mean what we say to a child, when what we say is important. When we don't, or when he cannot possibly understand what we say to him even if we do mean it, we are teaching him by so much that speech can be unsatisfying and somehow unpleasant, and that perhaps it is not always to be trusted because people can use it to keep us from knowing what they really feel and mean. When our actions tell a youngster one thing while our words seem to say something very different, he will mostly believe our actions and learn to be suspicious of what we say. Honesty is the best policy — but, because honesty is by no means simple, it is especially important that we be honest in making clear to children that we do not always know whether we are being honest with them or not. They should never be able to doubt, though, that we are trying to be.

There is more to be shared with our children, however, than the things we are sure they must learn before sundown and the bitter without which the sweet will be bland. There are warmth and laughter, and things that are silly, and odds and ends of wish and memory. There are the old jokes and riddles and all sorts of new surprises, and the joys of birthdays, and there is the sharing of family feelings on the holy days of the many faiths, and there is the monkey business of April Fools' Day, and the jolly bewitching of Halloween. The more experiences we share with our children the more we have to share with them in words.

Over the years I have offered to many mothers and fathers the rather simple suggestion that they make a practice of reading aloud to their children, especially at bedtime. The results, so far as I have been able to know them, have been wonderfully good. If you read your tike a story before you tuck him into bed you bring his day to a close and prepare him for a restful night in about as warmly pleasant a way as can be imagined. As he snuggles against you, listening

167

to you read just for him a delightful story, he associates the sounds of your voice with very nearly the nicest feelings he will ever know. In addition to all the other good that comes of this, you and your youngster acquire together from these stories read at bedtime a whole world of fact and fancy which you will share through all your days, and it will make talk between you endlessly. Your child gains words by the score, and a fabulous gallery of pictures in his head, and with them understandings and emotions that would never otherwise be his, and these will season delightfully the sense he will make and the pleasure he will find in his own speech.

After all, speech is like a wand, bringing back again the past we talk about, and it is most rewarding when the past it brings back is full of joy and wonder.

CHAPTER 11

How You Can Help Yourself

IF YOU are personally caught up in the problem called stuttering you are by no means alone. You are one in seven of every thousand, a vast company of over one million persons in the United States. Assuming the same ratio, there are more than a million stutterers in Russia, a third of a million in England, four million in China, and approximately twenty million among the nearly three billion men, women, and children in all the world.

As a member of this great company, would you say that the following brief description of your problem is reasonably accurate? You have learned to doubt that you can speak "fluently enough." You have learned to fear what might happen if you don't. Because of your doubt you expect to have trouble when you speak. Because of your fear you try to keep from having this trouble. In your effort to avoid it you proceed with caution, hesitantly, on the lookout for "difficult" words or sounds. If you feel that you are about to stutter, or that you already are stuttering, you try to stop, because you don't want to go on stuttering. But it takes an effort to stop, because you want very much to go on talking. It takes an effort to go on talking, however, because you are trying to stop so you won't continue stuttering. You feel as though you were being pulled apart by opposing forces in a tug of war. You feel, in varying degrees, tension and embarrassment, even a touch of anger and resentment perhaps, and a surge of determination, or an urge to vanish in thin air, and maybe a dash of foolishness—all rolled up into one complex experience that is as distressing as it is largely because it is so mysterious.

If that is your problem, then you have known in your life one special day of destiny, and doubtless you pray that there will be another. On the one that you have already known you were classified for the first time as a stutterer. On the other that is yet to be, you hope to break out of the category of "stutterer" and move happily into that of "normal speaker." This day, surely, you would hasten in all possible ways.

◄　◄　◄

How can you — not in the realm of hope and might-be, but in reality — deal effectively with your problem of stuttering and in the end solve it as fully as possible? If you are old enough to be chiefly on your own in doing what you can about the problem, you have much to gain by way of background information and understanding from a reading of the first ten chapters of this book. Because they are about the origins of stuttering, they speak directly to you concerning the fundamental nature of the problem. They provide you with a basis for making the most in a practical way of the explanations and recommendations in the pages that follow.

Valuable as the reading of a book can be, there are good reasons why you should also seek out a speech clinic and take advantage of the services it has to offer you. Through the American Speech and Hearing Association, 1001 Connecticut Avenue N.W., Washington 6, D.C., you can find out about clinical speech services available in your region. You can also address inquiries to your nearest university, as well as your state Department of Education. Your physician will be glad to assist you in locating appropriate clinical speech services. It is essential that you do your best to get the services you need — and to help yourself. It is reasonable to expect that you will help yourself by a careful study of these pages and a conscientious effort to apply what you learn from them. If you elect to do this, it is to be hoped that you will exercise your best judgment in adapting to your own circumstances — and, in some instances, perhaps disregarding — the advice you find here. This advice is unavoidably colored to some degree by my personal experience with the problem called stuttering. This experience has been extremely fortunate — the road from the severe stuttering I used to know to the speaking I do now has been an increasingly pleasant one. It has been one man's road, however, and the journey you would take may well follow another trail. Indeed, I shall tell you of many ways to the possible improvement of your speech. It would be best, even so, to work with a qualified speech clinician, if you can arrange to do this, in attempting to make use of the recommendations that follow.

Whether or not you go to a speech clinic, it will pay you to put together as best you can the story of the way your speech problem originated and developed to its present form. The facts that you are able to recall will help you to understand the things that have benefited you and those that have made your problem worse, and to see what you might better do differently now and in the future. You will gain even more value from admitting frankly that your memory is limited and that there are some facts you cannot recall — and others you are not sure about or do not understand very well. This will help you to approach your problem with an open mind and a readiness to learn all you can, instead of clinging to old ideas that are not likely to work any better in the future than they have in the past.

There are some basic questions about yourself that you might want to think about. These concern your more important relationships with other people, your feelings about yourself and your future, your main interests and likes and dislikes, your fears and worries, ambitions, hopes, and aspirations. How do you feel about your stuttering? What difference would it make to you — what you would do that would be different from what you are already doing — if you were to awaken in the morning and find your problem gone?

By thinking about these questions and answering them as well as you can you will become more understanding of yourself, more accepting or tolerant of the way you talk. You will come to feel more and more like talking. You will talk, therefore, more easily and fluently. You have felt for so long that when you stuttered your listeners were somehow critical or disapproving. You have more or less adopted what you supposed their attitude was, and so you have tended to be disapproving of yourself. You know that hasn't made it any easier for you to talk well. On the contrary, it has made speaking more difficult. It is not good for you to be critical and disapproving of yourself and of your way of talking. It is much better to be self-

171

accepting and self-approving. When you feel that you are doing the best you can you should feel a genuine acceptance of the best you can do. If you will do that, if you will be understanding of yourself and feel better about yourself and the way you talk — you will speak less uneasily and more spontaneously and smoothly. It is reasonable to expect, then, that you will improve steadily, with ups and downs, to be sure, but with a definite trend toward better and better and more enjoyable speech, if only you give yourself the benefit of warm self-acceptance and encouragement.

◄ ◄ ◄

The better your understanding of your speech problem, and of what you yourself are doing that complicates the problem, the more you can do to help yourself feel capable of dealing with it successfully. Here are some things to think about in order to gain a better understanding of what you call your stuttering. What sort of language do you use in talking about your problem? Are the questions you ask vague or down to earth? Do you talk mostly in generalities or do you usually try to make specific and descriptive statements about what you do when you stutter?

Do you talk or think mainly about your stuttering as something that happens to you — or as something that you yourself do? Do you take for granted that you *are* a "Stutterer," as though you were a native of Stutterania, perhaps, a special kind of being? Do you assume you *have* something or other inside you, such as a "tendency to stutter," or "nervousness" — or "Stuttering," like that, with a capital S, as though "it" might be a Something with a will of "its" own that comes and goes, and gets better and worse, as though you had no control over "it" or responsibility for "it."

It is much better for you to talk or think about what you *do*, rather than what you *are* or *have*. When you talk about what you *are* and what you *have* you tend to keep yourself from considering what you might *do* that would be an improvement over what you are *doing* now. If you tell yourself you *are* a kind of person — a Stutterer, for example, as though Stutterers were somehow in a basic way different from Normal Speakers — then you are likely to feel that there is nothing you can do about it: "The leopard can't change its spots." "If you don't have it you just don't have it." If you are in the habit of thinking and of saying things like that you are likely to tell yourself also "Once a Stutterer always a Stutterer" — and you might then go on to the depressing thought that there's really no hope for you. Or if there is, it is the wishful hope that Somewhere Sometime you will be lucky and find Someone who will take away, or drive away, what you *have* and transform you, as though by sorcery, from the Stutterer you *are* into the Normal Speaker you long to *be* One Day. Such wishfulness makes for dreams, particularly daydreams, about magical potions in the form of pills, or secret and mysterious Methods that can work Wonders. It does not encourage you to face up to the problem yourself and do something constructive about it here and now by your own efforts.

When, on the other hand, you talk about what you *do* that interferes with your speaking — such as pressing your lips together tightly, or holding your breath by tensing the muscles in your throat — you are more likely to see that you don't really have to do those things, and that you would talk more smoothly if you didn't. You can try, at least, to go ahead and talk without doing those things and find out what you do then. If you just talk, fine. When you do something else instead, like pressing your tongue against the roof of your mouth, you can sort of smile at yourself, as it were, and wonder what in the world you are doing that for. There is no need to scold yourself for doing it. There is much need not to scold but rather to be wholly accepting and understanding of yourself. And you have need, of course, to learn, to "get hep" to, just what it is you are doing, and why, and what your more desirable possibilities are.

You can ask yourself some very useful questions, therefore, such as, "Do I really have to tense up like that?" "What evidence do I have for saying that I have to do it?" "If there is no evidence that I need to hold my breath, what do I hope to gain by doing it?" "Does it help me to talk smoothly?" "Does it help me in any other way?" "Would I talk more smoothly if I just didn't do it at all?" "Would I talk more fluently and say what I want to say sooner if I were to do something else — for example, repeat the first part of the word a few

173

times easily, or just sort of stretch out or prolong the first sound of the word lightly and smoothly, in case I feel hesitant and don't seem to be ready to go ahead for a bit?" "And just what exactly is my reason for not feeling like going ahead for a bit?"

Talking and thinking about what you do, instead of what you assume you *are* and *have*, suggest all sorts of ways of *changing what you do*. It is nearly impossible, on the other hand, to see how you might change what you *are* or what you *have* — especially when you say you *are* a Stutterer and that what you *have* is a Something like a Disorder or a Condition that is Stuttering. And there is a very important difference, indeed, between thinking of yourself as a Stutterer and regarding yourself as a very much all right sort of person who sometimes does things that you or someone else may call "stuttering."

There is no need, of course, to call yourself names, such as "a Stutterer," at all. It is better just to describe as clearly as you can what it is you do when you talk easily and fluently, and just what it is you sometimes do — which you call stuttering — that prevents you from speaking easily and fluently. What you do you have learned to do. What you have learned to do that keeps you from speaking better than you do, you can unlearn. There is, to my knowledge, no physical reason why you can't learn to speak more easily and fluently than you do now. If that is the case, there is nothing to be gained by telling yourself you can't. There is ever so much that is good to be gained by telling yourself that you are not to be blamed for doing what you have unintentionally learned to do — and that you are fully capable of doing better and better and better, chiefly by wholeheartedly accepting the best you can do in the meantime.

It makes sense to get as well acquainted as you can with the good speaking you do — and with the fact that much of the time you speak very well indeed. When you are all alone you seldom or never do the things you call your stuttering, if you are like practically all the adult stutterers I have known. Moreover, you talk all right to your dog or your horse. You can read right along with the others in the congregation on Sunday mornings in church during responsive readings. And you can probably point to other sorts of speaking which you do normally, or to certain persons with whom you seldom or never experience discomfort in speaking. What is more, the greater part of your talking day in and day out, in the situations in which you hesitate and strain as well as those in which you don't, is made up of fluent speech rather than the apprehensive, tense, avoidant reactions you feel and think of as stuttering.

It is very good for you to understand clearly that the things you do that interfere with the normally easy flow of your speech are indeed things *you do* yourself. They do not *just happen to you*. The reason you find this hard to grasp is that whenever you tense up you do it so very suddenly, as a rule, practically before you know you've done it. It is easy to get the illusion that you had absolutely nothing to do with it. On top of that, you will swear that the only thing in the world you want to do is to go on with what you are trying to say — but that "the word just won't come out." Of course, if you stop to notice what you are doing — you are perhaps pressing your lips together very tightly, and that is not a very good way to go on talking! It's downright surprising, isn't it, to come to and discover that with all the effort you are putting forth you are mainly keeping your mouth tightly shut, when all the time you thought you were making a mighty effort to speak. It is very much as though in driving your car you were to press down harder and harder on the brake, thinking all the while that you were stepping on the gas.

Now, if in driving your car you did find that you had pressed down on the brake instead of the gas, it would be sensible to lift your foot, and then take it off the brake altogether before pressing gently on the gas. It doesn't take much effort to step on the gas; it takes much more to press down on the brake and hold it down. In driving a car, then, whenever you are exerting any noticeable effort, and your car begins to slow down or comes to a stop, you know that you are stepping on the brake and not on the gas.

Speaking is a good deal like that. When you seem to be wanting and trying to go forward, but at the same time are plainly stopped, it is sensible to stop straining, and just do, with no more effort than is called for, what comes next. It takes almost no effort at all to go forward, making one movement — or, rather, one flowing pattern of movements — after another in speaking. It takes considerable effort, however, to bring your speaking to a halt, or to hold back from beginning to speak when you want to talk. In speaking, then, as in driving, whenever you find that you are exerting any noticeable effort, and you begin to stall or come to a standstill, you know that you are trying for some reason to keep from talking, as well as trying to talk. When you try to do both at the same time you find yourself doing the things you think of as your stuttering.

What reason could you have for trying *not* to talk? I think you know the answer. You say you don't want to stutter, or to continue stuttering, and so you try to avoid the stuttering you expect, or to stop the stuttering that is "going on." You say "going on," because that is how it feels to you, as though it were going on all by itself, not as though you yourself were doing it. As though by instinct, or by reflex action, you act quickly, almost without knowing you are *doing* anything — or, as we say, "unconsciously." You act to avoid or to stop "the stuttering." So you act — and it turns out that what you avoid, or stop, or disrupt, is the activity necessary for speech.

The core of the truth is that in doing this you play an amazing trick on yourself. You do it so fast, and your motives and feelings and beliefs are such, that you are never likely to catch on to it unless someone runs it through in slow motion, as it were, and shows you just how you manage to fool yourself. If the following description is as successful as I hope it is, it will help to make reasonably clear just what you do.

Let us suppose that you are going to say, "Please pass the potatoes." You don't speak right up, though, because you are not sure you can say "potatoes." Maybe a little later. But the more you think about "potatoes" the more certain you become until finally you fully expect to stutter on "potatoes." You are strongly tempted, therefore, to go without potatoes. At the same time, you are hungry and you like potatoes. Besides, you have a lot of gumption, and you don't like to feel defeated. So, after a moment of conflict, you throw yourself to the mercy of your fate and say, "Please . . ." As you move on through "pass" and into "the" you prepare to avoid if possible the difficulty you feel certain you are going to have with "potatoes." You are resolved to try hard to say "potatoes" in spite of the stuttering that you feel sure is going to occur.

You do, indeed, try hard. And the stuttering you expected does, indeed, occur. What "occurs," that is, is that in trying to "keep from stuttering" in saying "potatoes" you exert effort, as if by instinct or by conditioned reflex. You do this by pressing your lips together very tightly. You sincerely believe that by doing this you will somehow manage to "force out the word as quickly as possible." You "force" very hard to overcome the stuttering you expect to "get in your way." And, sure enough, you "meet with resistance." You "have trouble." The "stuttering" you expected does turn out to be "difficult to handle." You did not succeed in avoiding "it," in spite of your avoidant effort, and now you have difficulty breaking through or out of "the block." You try harder. Precisely how do you do this? Why, to be sure, by pressing your lips more tightly together.

What you call your stuttering and your effort to avoid or to break out of "it" — these are one and the same thing! What is "holding the word in" is simply the effort that you are exerting to "force it out." What you call your stuttering and the things you are doing to avoid "it" are the same. What you call your stuttering and your effort to say "potatoes" in spite of "it" are not two things, but one only.

What you experience as your stuttering is what you do trying not to stutter again — or any longer. You will not "stutter" unless you try — in the ways you try — to avoid "stuttering," because what you do to avoid "it" is what you experience as your stuttering. The instant you stop doing what you do in trying not to stutter you stop doing everything that feels like stuttering.

There is still more to this incredible trick you play on yourself when you try not to stutter. It is built upon one of the most powerful and deceptive illusions you are likely ever to know. First, as we have seen, you expect to stutter — and because of what you do to keep from stuttering your expectation is proved correct. That is, you do the things that to you are stuttering. This strengthens your tendency to expect stuttering. That is, if you expect to "have trouble" saying a word, and then you do "have trouble," you will be still more inclined to expect to "have trouble" the next time you have to say that

177

word. And not only that word but also other words that seem to you to be like it — that begin with the same sound, for example, or that are about the same length, or that are to be spoken to the same sort of listener or in a similar situation, or with a like tone of voice, and so on. You will not expect difficulty in saying all such words every time you have to say them, of course. The number or proportion of them arousing your expectation of trouble will vary, for example, from situation to situation and from listener to listener. The main point is that you do learn to expect trouble, and the more often and the more painfully your expectancy is borne out, the more thoroughly you learn to expect trouble.

In the second place, you also learn more and more thoroughly to do the things you do in trying to avoid or stop what you call the stuttering — because you nearly always end up saying the word, or some word at any rate, and so you seem to succeed, after all. The illusion is, you see, that it was whatever you did that finally enabled you to say what you wanted to say, or at least to say something.

Because of this illusion of success, "finally getting the word out" serves to reinforce your tendency to do the same things again in an effort to "get the word out," or to "release yourself from the stuttering block." So, strange as it may seem when stated this way, if you press your lips together with great tension for a long time but then finally say "potatoes," you will tend to learn to press your lips together tightly whenever you have to say "potatoes." And you will learn to do this in saying many other words that are like "potatoes" because they begin with *p* or other lip sounds, or they are spoken at the dinner table, or to people who resemble your dinner companions, or are spoken under conditions of candlelight — provided you happened to be eating by candlelight sometime when you felt extreme distress saying "potatoes."

In other words, the behavior you call your stuttering is more or less self-perpetuating. It feeds on itself. The more you expect to stutter, and then do the things that to you are stuttering, the more you will expect to stutter, even though the stuttering you expect is only what you yourself do because you expect to stutter. The more you try one time — or the more times you try — to "force the word out in spite of the stuttering," perhaps by pressing the lips together very hard, and then finally say the word, the harder you will try again the same way — or the more often you will try — to "force the word out in spite of the stuttering." In other words, you learn the error of thinking that the stuttering against which you struggle is different from your struggle, when all the time the stuttering lasts only so long as you struggle against it — because your struggle and what you experience as your stuttering are one and the same.

You began to learn to do these things — without meaning to, of course, and without anyone else wanting you to — when you first were given to feel that something you were doing when you spoke was unacceptable and was therefore not to be done. If you are like nearly all others who think of themselves as stutterers, you were very young, probably around three, when you first started to feel that something about the way you were speaking was not all right. As you came to recognize that what seemed to be unacceptable to the important grownups you talked to were your hesitations and repetitions, you began to try not to hesitate and repeat sounds or words or phrases. At first, about all you felt, if indeed you were aware of anything at all, was a little holding back sometimes in speaking, and so you spoke just a bit more hesitantly. As your well-meaning listeners sensed this they got across to you somehow, mostly by means of subtle changes in their listening posture, facial expression, tone of voice, and the like, that they wished still more strongly that you wouldn't hold back or hesitate or repeat even more than you had been doing. In turn, you tried a little harder, and so you hesitated a bit more and began repeating a little tensely perhaps. In their turn, your important listeners seemed more concerned than ever, and so you were still more careful and tried still harder, and became more tense, and they grew more worried — and at some point along the way you acquired their way of thinking that what you were doing was stuttering and that what you were was a stutterer, and that it was bad to be a stutterer and that you should try not to stutter.

This learning process has been going on ever since — and here you are now, doing the things you have learned so well to do, under the illusion that what you call your stuttering and what you try so hard to do about it, or to control it, or avoid it, or break out of it, are two different things. But they are one and the same thing — and so the more you do what you take to be stuttering the harder you try to do something about "it," and the harder you try to do something about "it" the more you do of the things you take to be stuttering — so long, that is, as you think your stuttering is not something you do, but something about which you have to do something.

The illusion has a third peculiarly important effect: it tends to strengthen your feeling that what you call your stuttering really is something quite beyond your control, something that happens to you, not because of what you do but in spite of all you do to keep "it" from happening. The quality of the total experience causes you to think of what you call your stuttering as something aside from yourself, with a will of its own. The language you use in talking about "it" tends to be animistic — that is, you seem to be talking about animisms, or "gremlins," of one kind or another. You refer to your stuttering much as you would speak of a living thing. It comes and goes, you say, and gets better and worse of itself. You seem to be saying, indeed, that you are somehow possessed. You even talk about words that won't come out, as though the words had minds of their own and they themselves decided whether to come out or stay in. You say your tongue gets tense, as though it were not you who tensed your tongue, pressing it yourself against the back of your teeth. The illusion you express in these ways is that your stuttering is not of your own doing. You tend, therefore, to take for granted that it is a "disorder" of some sort, a "symptom" of something or other like a disease, or a "weakness," or an "instability." Under the spell of this way of thinking — and this sort of language — you see nothing to do but to contend with "the stuttering" as though "it" were an outside force, to try to control "it," to struggle against "it," to strive to talk in spite of "it." You do not see that what you speak of and think about in this animistic way as your stuttering is, in fact, something you do yourself — and that you can change what you do. As soon as you see this, you can see also some of the ways you can change what you do in order to improve the way you speak.

The illusion that what you call your stuttering is not of your own doing has a fourth profound consequence. You tend to make various personality adjustments — and maladjustments — on the basis of it. Thinking of what you call your stuttering as something for which you are not personally responsible, you quite naturally regard yourself as a disabled and handicapped person. You have a disorder, you say, an abnormal condition or characteristic that marks you as different from other people. You take for granted that you are a stutterer, a special kind of person, and a kind that no one wants to be. You tend to think about yourself in ways that keep you from realizing what a very worthwhile and acceptable person you are.

In one way or another you adjust to this notion you have of yourself. Most ways of adjusting to it are undesirable. There are, it is true, a few ways of reacting to it that do have their good points. The thought that you are a stutterer may fill you with a resolve to be more than just a stutterer, and so you may develop your talents in music, sports, or some kind of academic work, perhaps, with consequent achievements beyond what you might otherwise have known. This sort of motivation can be constructive, provided it does not drive you too hard or in ill-advised directions.

Another form of advantageous adjustment is that of using what you think of as your handicap as a means of cultivating your capacity to understand what a handicap means, not only to you but to other persons with other kinds of disadvantage as well. You can learn, for example, if you will, from being classified and dealt with as a stutterer what it feels like to belong to a minority group, because being reacted to as a stutterer is to some extent like being reacted to, not on your own merits as an individual, but as a white man in the Far East, or an Oriental or a Negro in a white culture, or as a "Foreigner," a "Stranger," an "Outlander," or any other "kind of person" who is assumed to be strangely different. If you can come through the experience of "being a stutterer" with a more ready understanding of your fellow human beings, you may conclude that it has been worth all the disadvantage you have known because of it. You are nearly certain to say, with deep sincerity, that you are grateful for the gifts brought you by distress — and so join the vast company who have in their varied ways found good fortune in adversity.

For the most part, however, if you think of yourself as a handicapped person you are likely to do some things because of this that can have various kinds of unfortunate effects. Indeed, what you call your stuttering is not your main handicap by any means.

In speaking one time before a convention of the National Society for Crippled Children and Adults — the Easter Seal Society — Louise Baker, author of the wise and delightful book *Out on a Limb,* told a story which I doubt has ever been forgotten by anyone who was in the audience that day. She used a crutch gracefully in walking to the rostrum, and she explained that when she was a little girl she had lost a leg in an encounter between her bicycle and an automobile. Her father was a clear-eyed realist who allowed that the fact she had lost a leg was no reason for treating her differently from her brothers and sisters. Whenever he thought she deserved a spanking he gave her one. A kindly neighbor lady, Mrs. Robinson, had an entirely different view of the matter, and did not hesitate to tell Louise that she did not agree at all with Mr. Baker's ideas of discipline. One day, Louise said, when she was about nine, she came home from an afternoon of kindness and cookies at dear old Mrs. Robinson's house, thumped her little crutch across the living room to her father's easy chair, and said, "Daddy, Mrs. Robinson says she doesn't think you ought to spank a poor little handicapped girl like me." Mr. Baker looked for a long moment with a very steady gaze into her upturned accusing eyes and then in slow, firm tones replied, "You go back and tell Mrs. Robinson that that's not where you're handicapped!"

The stuttering that you call your handicap — that's not where you're handicapped. Your major handicap stems from the fact that you labor under the illusion that you are a handicapped person, because you believe that your stuttering is not your personal responsibility, that it is something that happens to you rather than something you do yourself. You say you "can't help it," and so you feel helpless. While it is true that you can make adjustments to this illusion that may have good effects — just as an occasional oyster creates a pearl in reacting to the irritation caused by a grain of sand — your main tendency, like that of most oysters in response to most grains of sand, is likely to be unproductive, or worse. You may, for example, not attempt to do many things that you could do. You may feel a little sorry for yourself. You may tell yourself that speaking is difficult, and situations in which speaking is necessary are hazardous, and so stay home instead of going to the party, or not attempt to go to college, or not apply for a job you might very well be able to fill successfully. In general, you may be inclined, if you are not objective and thoughtful, to adjust to your illusion by selling yourself short.

If you do not sell yourself short, there are still other ways of working your way into trouble. One of these is by refusing to admit that you have any problem at all. You may even go to the extreme of trying to pass yourself off not as a potential but as an actual normal speaker, although regarding yourself all the while as a stutterer. In doing this, you are almost certain, of course, to deceive yourself much more than anyone else — like the stuttering freshman in college who told his classmates he was not going to try out for the debate team because he was too tall. And then there was the other freshman who tried out for the debate team, but indignantly rejected the coach's suggestion that he go to the speech clinic, where he might have been helped to improve enough to perform effectively as a debater.

If you are like nearly all the other adult stutterers I have known, you create — without meaning to, of course — a major share of any adjustment difficulties you may have, by trying to cover up, conceal, or disguise the fact that you talk the way you do, and that you think and feel the way you do about it. In trying to accomplish this ill-advised purpose — which, of course, you practically never accomplish anyway — you sometimes withdraw from social situations in which you could often find pleasure, enlightenment, and friendship. In the classroom, and elsewhere as well, you give no answers, or even wrong answers, when you could give yourself and others the benefit of good answers. You do not ask questions when they would, in some situations, be much more illuminating than the answers others are quick to give. You sometimes create the impression of aloofness, or unfriendliness, or stupidity when you are in reality sociable, friendly, and well informed.

In our clinic there was once a young lady who gave the appearance of being extremely unresponsive to other people — but now and then she would ride the train to the next town, wait there in the station for a few hours, and then ride the next train back, because, as she confided to her clinician, she deeply enjoyed being with other people. She couldn't bear to have them think that "she was a stutterer," however, and so she preferred strangers, with whom she did not feel a need to talk, to friends or acquaintances who would expect her to join in their conversation. There are many seemingly shy and retiring persons who are warmly outgoing, but their friendly impulses are frustrated by their unfortunate, and unnecessary, notion that to be themselves is to be rejected. They would gain rewards beyond their most unfettered dreams from learning that if they are to know the deep satisfactions of feeling that they are being understood they must make themselves understandable. This they can never do by self-disguise but only through self-revelation.

One of the saddest forms of poor adjustment to the experience of "being a stutterer," and in the long run the most serious, is that of not taking advantage of available information, reading material, and clinical services. It is not that this is peculiar only to persons who regard themselves as stutterers. There are millions of people with various reasons for needing help who are gravely handicapped by their failure to seek the help they need, or to make good use of it once they find it — or it is brought to them. They have never learned one of the greatest lessons that any child can ever be taught: *To be helped one must be helpable, to be taught one must be teachable.* Like the priceless sentiment of the poet Ovid, "To be loved one must be lovable," this lesson points up a basic principle of all human relationships, which is that they are not one-way relationships, they work both ways, they are interactions.

To say this is to believe it. We know it must be true. Yet — we often speak as though we disbelieved every word of it. We talk as though we expected to be taught by our teachers rather than to learn *with* them. We seem all too often to think doctors are supposed to keep their patients well, or when they are sick to make them well, as though it were enough for the patient to be patient.

184

Dr. Lee Edward Travis told me one time of a mother who telephoned to say that his suggestion that she not be critical of her Willie's speech and that she show him more affection had worked fine, and little Willie was talking very well now, so would it be all right if she went back to treating him normally again!

To be helped you must be helpable, and to be helpable you must work with those who are trying to work with you. Other persons can hardly do more than make it possible for you to help yourself. I can only write this book, for example. The publisher and booksellers can make it available to you. But you have to read it and work at trying to understand it, and do your best to apply what you learn from it to your specific needs for improvement in your particular situation.

The same will be true if you go to a speech clinic. Those who work there can only make helpful information, instruction, and counseling available to you. But they cannot feel your feelings, think your thoughts, or move with your muscles. They cannot do your talking. You and you alone can do these things. Only you can possibly take final, working responsibility for what you feel, or think, or say, or do. Only you can change your usual ways of doing things, or speaking, or thinking, or feeling.

If you understand clearly that you must help yourself, and that you can, you will be likely to talk freely with others — professional persons and family and friends — about your problem and what you might do and are doing about it, and why. This will help them very much to be as helpful to you as they would like to be. What, for example, do you prefer to have your listeners do while you are struggling to begin speaking or to go on speaking to them? Your answer may well be that it doesn't matter much what they do so long as they manage to make you feel that they respect you and are friendly or positive in their feelings toward you. Whatever your answer is, your listeners would be sincerely interested in it. You will find that nearly everyone is all for you, eager to do "the right thing," interested in your problems and in your progress. They will want to be helpful, and the ones who will help you the most are those who seem to take for granted that you are doing the best you know how to do, and so they take you as you are and by doing that they make you feel a little taller.

It is good for you to feel a little taller. It is best that you feel a warm acceptance of yourself as a person. You have every reason to feel that you are physically and in all other ways capable of speaking normally as other folks do — and that if you don't sometimes the reasons are not to be held against you. The reasons are that you learned — through no fault of yours, or of anyone else for that matter, but rather in spite of the best of intentions by everyone concerned — to doubt that you could speak smoothly enough and to be afraid of not doing so. It is good for you to feel perfectly capable of working your way out of your unnecessary doubts and fears — and to set about doing it.

❧   ❧   ❧

What, then, can you do to help yourself? Here are some of the more basic suggestions that follow from all that I have said.

First: *Pay much more attention to your normal speech than to what you think of as your stuttering. Cultivate increasingly the feelings and attitudes and ways of thinking that go with normal speech. Be warmly accepting of your speech and of yourself as a person.*

Saturate your consciousness with the fact that you exert practically no effort at all in speaking normally. Do this in part by talking and reading aloud a great deal when you are alone, or to your dog, or to any persons to whom you speak or read well, or in any situations where you do not do what you call your stuttering. Do some of this speaking and reading while watching yourself in a mirror, seeing with your own eyes that your normal speech not only feels free of tension but also looks effortless and pleasant. If you have access to a tape recorder or an office dictation machine, you should speak into it and then listen to your speech. You should do this when you are alone, or to one or more listeners with whom you speak smoothly, and then listen over and over again to yourself speaking, or reading aloud, normally. You should listen to recordings of your normal speech until it sounds right and natural to you, until it sounds like you. It is much to your advantage to learn that your speech feels,

186

looks, and sounds good — when you don't do the things, which you call your stuttering, that interfere with it.

Pay more attention to the speech of others whom you regard as normal speakers. There are two main things to notice about their speech. One is that it is not perfectly fluent; the other is that it usually seems to be effortless. It is particularly important for you to observe that even when a normal speaker is fumbling for words, saying uh uh uh, stumbling over the pronunciation of a word, or repeating repeating re repeating like this or like li like this, he doesn't seem to be bothered especially, or to "fight it," or to try to keep from doing what he is doing, and he doesn't "tense up." He seems to be as free of tension or strain when saying uh uh, or repeating words or even syllables, as he is in talking straight along with no bobbles.

It is good for you to realize that much of your own hesitating and fumbling in speaking is like that of other folks. If you are like most other speakers who think of themselves as stutterers, you tend to suppose that unless your speech flows as smoothly as a meadow brook you are not talking normally. Actually, many of your disfluencies are like those of normal speakers, and are so regarded by them when they hear you. You will recall that in the study by Dr. Curtis Tuthill, referred to near the end of Chapter 2, adult stutterers as well as college freshmen who were normal speakers and knew nothing in particular about speech pathology listened to recorded samples of speech and marked what they regarded as "stuttered words" on mimeographed copies of the material. The stutterers had much "longer ears" than the other listeners. They marked roughly 40 per cent more words as "stuttered" than did the freshmen. This means that if these stutterers had adopted the same definition of "stuttering," or "stuttered word," as the normal speakers were using, they would have immediately "stuttered" 40 per cent less — and *without speaking any more fluently*!

There is an exceedingly important lesson for you in these facts. You will remember that Dr. Dean Williams has reported (see Chapter 10) that when parents are asked to listen for the *normal* hesitations and repetitions in their children's speech, they don't hear as many that sound like "stuttering" to them. They come to feel, there-

187

fore, that their youngsters are talking better, with all the benefits that follow for both them and their children from this "change of ear." Just so, if you will begin to pay much more attention to those things about your own speech that you call normal, including your breaks in fluency that are normal, you are almost certain to feel better about the way you are speaking. The good effects of feeling better about it will add up to greater confidence, more enjoyment of speaking, more responsiveness and spontaneity in talking to other people, and a better feeling about yourself generally.

Listen more attentively and with a sense of evaluation to speakers on radio and television. Try to "feel along with them as they speak." When you are by yourself and can talk without doing what you call your stuttering, try talking like your favorite speakers, imitating them, getting the feel of what their normal speaking is like as best you can. If you can listen to radio or TV speakers at times when there is no one else around — or when you are with your speech clinician, or a helpful friend — try to say everything the speaker says, keeping up with him as closely as possible, and doing your best to duplicate his voice and expressiveness. This is called shadowing. It is a good way to practice as nearly as you can what normal speakers do when they talk. You will be struck, of course, by the lack of effort, the absence of any holding back of the sort that feels like stuttering, and the general easiness and "swinging along" feeling of it. You will also be impressed many times by the number of repetitions and other hesitations that are normal and wholly acceptable. One of the very most important things you will learn is that the best of human speech has about it the feel of forthrightness, of basic honesty and sincerity. It seems to be the sound of a person ringing true. You will notice that in this sort of speech there may be much of the slowness and hesitation of thoughtfulness, but there is none of the tension of self-rebuke, or the holding in that expresses fear of what the listener might think of the manner of speech.

Another kind of activity which will help you develop the feel of normal speech is that of reading aloud in chorus with your clinician or a friend who speaks normally. You will be able to do this quite readily. After you have done this awhile, you can ask your partner to stop reading and see how far you can go on alone. As soon as you tense up and stop yourself your partner can start reading aloud again at that point and you will be able to read along with him again. You will be able to read along with your partner even when the two of you are reading different materials, and you will want to try this, not only for the fun of it, but also to reinforce in this way the conviction that you are fundamentally a normal speaker, with no physical reason for having to do the things you call your stuttering. What may impress you most of all is that you can read fluently in chorus even with another stutterer, who will, of course, read fluently at the same time in chorus with you!

You may find it particularly helpful in getting the feel of how fully capable you are of normal speech to practice reading aloud or speaking as fast as you possibly can and still be understood. If you are like most stutterers you tend to speak and to read aloud more slowly than most normal speakers do, and so you are thoroughly used to the feel of relatively slow "heel-dragging" speech. You will probably hesitate and strain much less than usual, or even not at all, when you try to read or speak as rapidly as possible. In the bargain you will be cultivating feelings opposite to those of holding back and of excessive cautiousness in speaking. You will be getting to know more clearly what normal speech — your own normal speech — feels like.

You will find it a good idea, too, to talk with your clinician, or with members of your family, or friends, finding out what it seems like to them to speak normally. I think you will be surprised to find that they are hardly aware of just what it is that they do when they speak. Ask them to tell you precisely how they say "Massachusetts," for example! The fact that they won't be able to tell you is part of the reason they say it so easily. Part of your difficulty, perhaps, is that you take for granted that the *m* sound is hard to make, and that in order to make it there are certain things you have to be careful to do — such as pressing the lips together tightly for a while! You will benefit from observing — as though you were noticing it for the first time in your life — that your friends who speak smoothly don't press their lips together strenuously for a while before they say "Massachusetts" and other m words. You may be moved to wonder, as you have never wondered before, why you do. It will be good for you to discover that you just don't have any very solid answer to that question. This will hasten the day when you will no longer keep yourself from saying words by pressing your lips firmly together, or by doing other things that keep you from doing the smooth and easy speaking of which you arc capable.

Another important fact you will learn from your friends who speak normally is that they are by no means free of all anxieties and uneasiness when they are speaking. Most of them will tell you that they suffer at least a little from stagefright. It bothers them to ask the boss for a raise, to make certain telephone calls, to recite in school, to talk to a strange girl (or young man), or to important people, or to very nearly anyone on certain formal occasions, perhaps. They do not always feel sure of themselves or of what they have to say. They are sometimes reluctant to speak, doubtful of their wisdom, their rights, their taste, or their judgment. Now, you tend to take for granted that when you feel any fear or uneasiness about speaking, you are going to "stutter." Your friends don't "stutter" — they don't tighten up, jam the tongue up against the roof of the mouth, for example, and keep themselves from talking — when they feel uneasy and afraid. The extremely important lesson you have to learn from them is that you too, as well as they, can start, or continue, talking even when you feel afraid or uneasy about speaking. Many an actor has spoken his opening lines while all but frozen with fear. What you call your "fear of stuttering" does not really make it necessary for you to press your lips together tightly, or hold your breath, or do anything else that will interfere with your speech. It is especially good for you to find out that at any given moment you are able to do the next thing to be done in speaking — that is, to go ahead and speak — even at those times when you feel you can't.

In these ways, and in others that your clinician may suggest or that you may figure out for yourself, you can weaken and, it is to be hoped, finally destroy your feelings of doubt about your basic ability to speak normally. A major part of your program of improvement consists of demonstrating to your complete satisfaction that you can talk. By accomplishing this you will discover that when you don't speak easily and with normal fluency — and normal hemmings and hawings and stallings and stumblings — the reason is that you are doing other things instead, such as pressing your lips together tightly or holding your breath by tensing the muscles in your throat, that interfere with your speech. Since you learned to do these things in the first place, for reasons that seemed good at the time, you can now unlearn them, because you can no longer see any good reasons for doing them.

◄   ◄   ◄

Second: *Pay enough attention to the things you do that interfere with your normal speech, the things you do that you call your stuttering, that is, to understand that they are unnecessary and to change or eliminate them.*

You can work at carrying out this recommendation with the help of your speech clinician or a friend, or by yourself. You must be very clear what you are about when you do this. You are not to dwell on the mistakes you make in a spirit of self-criticism. You are not to feel badly because you make mistakes; on the contrary, you are to feel hopeful because you can correct them. In general, they are the sorts of errors you are not so likely to make if you recognize that they are, indeed, errors you make rather than mysterious "blockages" or "breakdowns" that happen to you, and that you have a good deal to do with just how you go about making the errors, or with whether or not you make them at all. No one can fairly blame you for making mistakes that you have learned through no fault of your own, and you should not blame yourself. It is highly commendable to recognize them frankly for the mistakes they are, to acknowledge them as your own, and to do what you can about them. You can be sure that others will think well of you if you do this — and it is altogether right that you should feel due admiration for yourself as you set about the important task of learning to speak better and more smoothly by changing and eliminating the things you are doing that keep you from talking as well as you can.

A particularly basic procedure is to talk or read aloud until you do something you call your stuttering, and then observe closely what

191

you are doing. Do it again immediately in order to get a better notion of just how you did it. Do it again, and perhaps again. Then do it again, but differently in some way. Do it more strenuously or for a longer time. Do it more easily. Change the way you do it; repeat the first part of the word easily and simply, or prolong the first sound of the word in a leisurely sort of way. The point of changing what you do is to break up your long established feeling that your stuttering happens to you, that you "can't help it," that it is not of your own doing. One of the most effective ways to weaken this feeling is to do deliberately, on purpose, what you call your stuttering. Get the feel of *doing* it. Then, in order to weaken still more the deep feeling you have that you can't do anything about it, *change* it, do it differently. Do it in many different ways, one after the other. Finally, say the word normally, without doing anything like your stuttering reactions at all. Say it again easily and smoothly. Again. And again.

This basic procedure can be elaborated and made more effective in a number of ways. One of these ways is to do it while observing what you are doing in a mirror. This simply helps to make obvious that what you call your stuttering is something that you are doing. It enables you to observe more carefully what you are doing and just how you are doing it. You see more clearly in a mirror what you can do to change what you do when you say you are stuttering. And the mirror sharpens your sense of the difference between stuttering in your usual way, or in some modified form, and speaking normally without doing anything to interfere with your basic speech activity.

Another way to add to the effectiveness of the procedure is to use a tape recorder. It is possible to observe your speech, and the things you do to interfere with it, much more objectively when you are listening to the playback of a tape recording of it. By using a tape recorder you tend to learn faster that your stuttering is, indeed, your own doing, and that the changes you can make in what you do are very substantial. You can practice making what you call your stuttering sound different in as many ways as possible — just as with a mirror you can practice making it look different in a great variety of ways.

There are two other useful things you can do with a tape recorder.

One of these is that you can shadow your own speech as you listen to it. You will recall what was said a few pages back about shadowing the speech of normal speakers on radio or TV, or "live," trying to say everything they say as quickly as possible after they have said it. By doing this while listening to a tape recording of your own speech, you become more conscious of what you do when you stutter, and when you speak normally — and of the difference between them — than you are likely to in any other way.

You will get more value from this basic procedure, with or without a mirror or tape recorder, if you carry it on in connection with another fundamental method, a sort of question and answer game that you can play with others or by yourself.

What you do is to talk or read aloud until you "are stuttering." Pay attention then to what you are doing. Hold it. Prolong it. Keep doing it. Observe it. It is likely to be something that you are doing with some degree of effort or tension, like tensely dragging out or prolonging the first sound of a word, s . . . uch as that, or repeating the first part of the word with effort, su su su such as that, or pressing the lips together firmly, or jamming the tongue tightly against the back of the front teeth or the roof of the mouth, or clamping the jaws tightly shut, or holding the breath by shutting off the passageway between the vocal folds by tensing the throat muscles, or some combination of these or other interfering activities.

Now, your speech clinician or a friend can help you by asking you — or you can ask yourself — precisely what you are doing. This is a question to be answered very carefully, with descriptive detail. Then you should ask yourself why you were doing what you were doing. Did you think you had to for some basic physical reason? Or for some other kind of reason? Do you have any scientific evidence for the reasons you give?

What specifically did you hope to accomplish by doing these things? Did you think you would say the word you wanted to say more easily, or sooner, or better, by doing them? Did you do these things in an effort to keep from stuttering? Would you have stuttered if you had *not* done these things? If you answer yes to this question, what do you mean by "stutter"? What evidence do you have?

If you had not done the things you observed yourself doing when you felt that you were stuttering, would you probably have spoken better, more smoothly, easily, and expressively, or less so? If you do not do these things in the future, do you think you will "stutter" less or more or not at all? Would you speak normally or satisfactorily if you did not do these things? If not, why not? If so, then what reason do you have for doing them at all?

By using this "what are you doing — why are you doing it — how would you speak if you didn't do it?" routine carefully, thoughtfully, kindly, and often enough, you are likely to learn, I think, sooner and more thoroughly than you might otherwise that the doubts, fears, tensions, and related reactions that you call your stuttering are neither necessary nor helpful. Indeed, without them you speak all right. It is an exercise that encourages you strongly to develop the conviction that you are basically a normal speaker — and that what you call your stuttering is something you do that you have learned and that you have every right to do, therefore, but that you don't need to go on doing when you have unlearned old feelings and ways of thinking and learned new ones. It helps to make clear that your stuttering is simply the things you do trying to avoid what you think of as stuttering, and that there is no stuttering to avoid if you do nothing to avoid it. It leads you, therefore, to wonder why, after all, you should try to keep from doing something that you will not do anyway if you don't try to keep from doing it. It tends to clarify your thinking, to improve your understanding of what you can do and should do, and it helps you, for these solid reasons, to feel more confident, and to accept yourself more completely.

⁌ ⁌ ⁌

Third: *Do more talking.*

This is a deceptively simple suggestion that needs a bit of explanation. Obviously, it is not meant, for example, that you should make a "talking pest" of yourself. It is not desirable to start needless or unpleasant arguments or to muddy the waters of discussion just for the sake of making talk. The best kind of talking for your purposes is that which you do in the course of being a good neighbor, of attending to your business or sharing your hobbies and interests, being a responsible citizen, a good roommate or club member, a pleasant and helpful member of your family, or a responsive friend. The bedrock consideration is that from now on you are to make a special point of not avoiding the talking that is yours to do in the ordinary course of daily living, the talking you would have been doing more fully all along had you not been holding back because of the way you have felt about what you call your stuttering.

The basic suggestion is that you begin to act as fully as possible as though you regarded yourself as a normal speaker. I say "as fully as possible" because you are dealing with a learning process. It is not to be expected that you will completely change your talking ways "all at once and nothing first." As you learn more and more, however, to think of yourself as a normal speaker, you will feel more and more like wanting to talk, and you will do more and more talking. The point of the recommendation is simply that such learning is to be achieved by working at it consistently and thoughtfully.

A principle that is fundamental in this learning is that success breeds confidence and, therefore, more success. It pays accordingly to put considerable stress on doing a good deal of speaking in the situations where you do well and enjoy talking. A practical way to do this to a limited extent is to read aloud to members of your family, or to friends, whenever you can. It is also a good idea, I think, to read aloud, preferably at least a few minutes each day, when you are by yourself, reading as expressively as you can.

There are probably certain situations, or kinds of speaking, that you tend especially to avoid. These may be telephoning, for example, or making introductions, asking for road information at service stations, or taking part in classroom discussions. You should aim to increase the amount of talking you do in such situations. You might begin to break down your fear of the telephone, for example, by calling your speech clinician if he is agreeable, or a friend, once or twice a day. You can use the telephone to answer certain want ads, preferably those in which you have at least some interest. As you can bring yourself to it, you will benefit from doing more and more of your personal and business communicating by telephone. As you lose

195

your fear of the telephone and come to enjoy using it, doubtless you will go beyond the calls that seem necessary or time-saving to doing a reasonable amount of telephoning that is mainly sociable. In this way you will use the telephone to keep more closely in touch with your friends, and you will gain pleasures and benefits far beyond those to be counted only in terms of "speech practice."

It would be difficult, indeed, to overstate the value to be gained through talking more with more people in more situations. What is being suggested is not pointless or "nuisance" talking, or mere talking for the sake of talking. What is being recommended is alert, friendly, interested, engaging responsiveness to other people. There is value for you in a wholesome desire to share your rewarding interests and your information when it would appear to be of use to someone else, to give your judgment and advice when they are wanted, or when they would be possibly helpful, or at least not inappropriate.

You need not wait to achieve a great deal of speech improvement before making a point of being more responsive in these ways to other people. You can do much to reverse the vicious circle of doubt-fear-tension-withdrawal-more doubt, etc., which you know only too well, and develop instead a benevolent circle of responsiveness-confidence-spontaneity-greater ease in speaking-more responsiveness, etc. Within limits, friendliness builds friendliness and confidence feeds on its own fruits. It is fully as true that nothing succeeds like success as it is that nothing fails like failure.

It is a sound rule, therefore, when applied within the boundaries of common sense, of course, that the more talking you do the better. In doing more talking in your daily rounds, it is a good idea to apply as consistently as you can everything you learn as you go along about the basic fact that your stuttering is something you do yourself. It is something you can do, therefore, in different and more simple and less effortful ways, so long as you do it at all, and with practice and thoughtful reflection and warm self-acceptance, you can in due time acquire the feelings and attitudes that make for normally smooth and easy speech.

All around you there are opportunities to practice speaking with the new feelings and ways of thinking through which you will tend to speak ever more easily, smoothly, and effectively — and with ever more enjoyment. Professional speech clinicians can help you take advantage of these opportunities by giving you essential information, instruction, and counseling. Your family, teachers, and friends can give you their moral support and cooperation and their time. By doing all you can to make the most of your opportunities for practice and improvement you stand to gain increasingly the rich rewards of self-realization.

❧ ❧ ❧

Everything that has been said up to this point leads to one final recommendation.

Fourth: *Work at "being a normal speaker."*

Just as the last recommendation, to do more talking, may have appeared to be deceptively simple, so this one may seem to be peculiarly vague. How do you "be a normal speaker" except by "speaking normally"? The point is that your task is not merely that of learning to speak differently but also that of learning — and of enabling others — to feel differently about you as a speaker and as a person.

You have had a reputation as a stutterer. Other people have made demands on you accordingly. They have expected you, for example, to participate or not participate in school activities, or in parties and other social events, in accordance with their concept of you as a stutterer. In some instances they have made excuses for you if you did not do well in activities in which you had to speak — and sometimes even in those not requiring speech. Likewise, they may have given you undue credit at times for quite ordinary accomplishments, thinking that you had done very well "for a stutterer."

The humorist Artemus Ward, speaking one time with this general sort of attitude, said, "I knew a man out in Oregon who didn't have a tooth in his head, not a tooth in his head, and yet that man could play the bass drum better'n any man I ever knew!" I have sometimes heard a stutterer lauded, with the same tones of misplaced wonder, for playing the clarinet splendidly or doing a fine job as a third baseman.

Your counselors and your parents may have taken your "being a stutterer" into account in various ways, not always realistically or with an eye to your good points and your capacity for growth, in advising you about school courses or your vocational future. Doubtless also your friends have many times changed a story, or refrained from telling a joke at all, or from singing "K-K-K-Katy," or in other ways "watched their tongues," because they thought of you as a "stutterer" and did not want to offend you. Only your very best friends would have told you, for example, about the fellow who was asked by a stutterer, with much strenuous repetition, how to get to the "li li li library." The man who was asked did not answer. The stutterer struggled through his question again. This time the man not only refused him the courtesy of a reply but actually turned and walked away from him. An outraged bystander accosted the fellow and demanded to know why he had not had the decency to tell the stutterer how to find the library. With palms upturned in a gesture of helplessness, the man explained, "Do you wuh wuh wuh want me to get poh poh poked in the nose?"

As far as other people have been concerned, you have not only talked in certain ways but you have also "been a stutterer." You have now to work, therefore, at "being" the sort of person others will think of less and less as a "stutterer" and more and more as a "normal speaker" — or, where speaking is concerned, as "just like anyone else."

Not only have you had a reputation; you have also had a self-image. You live from day to day and minute to minute with a certain conception or picture of yourself, of "who" you are and "what" you are. To the degree that you take for granted that you "are a stutterer" you do not readily think of yourself as "being a normal speaker." You are more or less like your family and friends, therefore, in the way you take the fact that you "are a stutterer" into account in making decisions from day to day about dating, or taking part in school activities, or civic affairs, or in planning — or not planning — your future. You, too, tend to make allowances for "being a stutterer" — not always necessarily for what you actually do when you speak, but for "being the kind of person you take yourself to be" — in excusing yourself for doing certain things halfheartedly or not at all. You, too, have told yourself, and others as well, perhaps, that you had done pretty well "for a stutterer," when as a matter of fact you could have done better. You are now undertaking, therefore, the job of remodeling the image or notion you have of yourself. You are going to work at "being" the sort of person that not only others but you also, and you especially, will think of less and less as a "stutterer" and more and more as a "normal speaker" — or, where speaking is concerned, as "just like anyone else."

You can make a start toward re-making yourself by answering, alone or with the aid of your clinician or a helpful friend, this very basic question that has been mentioned before: What difference would it make to you if you were to awaken tomorrow morning and find that you no longer "were a stutterer"? What would you do that you have not been doing? What have you been doing that you would no longer do? What old attitudes would you discard? What new interests would you cultivate?

When you have made your answers — act on them. There is no good reason to wait until tomorrow morning to begin acting *as best you can* as though you "were a normal speaker." Would you talk to more people? Then go ahead. Talk to as many as you can bring yourself to approach. Would you recite in your classes? Then make the best beginning you can muster. Would you go out with girls — and do you have a particular girl in mind? Ask her for a date, if not immediately, then as soon as you can talk yourself into doing it. But start immediately to talk yourself into it. If you are a girl and there is a boy you like, start being nice to him. If he doesn't ask you for a date, don't let the reason be that you didn't do your part — properly, of course, in good taste, but clearly enough to get your message across. If you "were not a stutterer" would you want to become a teacher, or a nurse, or a doctor, or a business executive? Then start thinking about it seriously. Talk to a vocational counselor if you can. If you can't, ask your librarian to help you find some reading materials about your favorite field of work. Learn all you can as objectively as possible about your abilities, and think realistically about your vocational future. In these and other ways take the steps you

— and only you — can take to move out of your castle of daydreams into the real world of planning and learning and working toward genuine goals.

If only you "were a normal speaker," would you, in the words of the popular song, accentuate the positive? Then go ahead and accentuate it. Cultivate your constructive interests and your talents. Start your music lessons now. Begin to sing, to rhumba, join a bowling team, learn to play bridge, take a course in Russian or Spanish, join a camera club, an investment group, go to night school, invite Joe to lunch and take Bill fishing with you, go in for golf or tennis, study salesmanship or accounting or electronics. Start doing the things you have wanted to do. There is no need to wait until you "are a normal speaker."

Do you wish you could talk to groups the way your friends do? At the beginning of the next school term sign up for a course in public speaking. Or read the want ads and find a job selling something from house to house. Or offer your services in selling Christmas trees for the local Optimist Club, or tickets to the upcoming Policemen's Dance. If you don't think you're ready to do anything like this, go to a speech clinic if you aren't already attending one, or practice harder, in any event, to modify the things you do that you call your stuttering, to test your ability to talk without doing these things, and to improve your speaking in every way you can. Work toward making yourself ready to take a public speaking course or a house-to-house selling job, or some other assignment in which you can act as much as possible as though you "were a normal speaker."

Accentuate the positive in the way you think and talk about yourself and others. What about you is admirable? Don't keep it a secret — don't brag, just admit it. What's your good news today? Tell it. What do you enjoy doing? Share your pleasures. Who are the persons you like or admire? Talk about them. Better yet, say everything good you can about those you don't like very well.

I am not advocating that you be a Pollyanna or a goody-good. It is only that if you are like most stutterers I have known, you stress the negative about yourself and other people and the world around you more than the objective facts warrant. You do a lot of suffering thinking about your suffering. You could have a lot more fun than you're having by talking more about the fun you're having.

I am not saying that you have nothing to complain about. I don't know whether or not you're being underpaid, or overworked, mistreated, or yammered at. I am saying that if you are, you should face up to the situation and do everything you can to improve it, and devote no more time than is necessary to dwelling on how awful it is. I simply think you should spend all the time you can getting to know your strong points, your opportunities, and the people who either have no desire to handicap you or who want to help you go where you want to go and be what you want to be. There is no life so dismal that it cannot be made yet more dismal by constant complaining about how dismal it is. Just so, it is our appreciation of even the least of good fortune that makes it better still.

¶ ¶ ¶

There is a final note of forewarning to be sounded. As you accept more and more of the advantages — and the responsibilities — of "being a normal speaker," you will want to be prepared to discover that the difference between the person you are now and the person you are becoming may not turn out to be as great as you have supposed it would be. There are two main reasons for this. The first is that you may come to believe that it is not as bad to "be a stutterer" as you have thought. The second is that you may decide that it is not as good to "be a normal speaker" as you have imagined. After all, among the differences you would face if you were to find tomorrow morning that you no longer "were a stutterer" would be the loss of certain kinds of sympathy and special consideration and the use of stuttering as an alibi. The sympathy and special consideration are nearly always misplaced, of course, and do you more harm than good, but even so you have learned to depend on them at least a little, and so you would miss them at first. Stuttering is not really any good to you as an alibi either, but again you would need to adjust to the fact that you no longer would have it available. You would also find that "being a normal speaker" means the taking on of certain responsibilities that you have not always been shouldering. Besides, after you have become a normal speaker you would look much as you do now. You would have no greater mental capacity than you now possess. You would be no taller or stronger or swifter. About many things you would think and feel quite the same as you always have. Nor would you be without problems of various kinds. Indeed, the life of a normal speaker can even be terribly hard, surprising as that may seem to you now without further reflection. Moreover, some words that are spoken fluently, even eloquently, cause profound anguish, while some words that are spoken with much strain and hesitation bring joy to all who hear them.

Sobering as these reflections may be, they do not mean that you will ever be likely to feel that it is better to "be a stutterer" than to "be a normal speaker." They are intended only to forestall the disappointments that could be yours if your memories were too forlorn and your anticipations too glorious. Meanwhile, it is, of course, a part of our most ancient wisdom that to be human is to speak. The more you come to know the joy of speaking, the more richly you will share the gift of your humanity.

INDEX

Index

205

CPSIA information can be obtained
at www.ICGtesting.com
Printed in the USA
BVHW060248040120
568548BV00016B/141/P

9 780816 660391